Ultrasound Imaging
for Rehabilitation
of the
Lumbopelvic Region

With great appreciation to all my teachers, past, present and future

For Elsevier:

Publisher: Heidi Harrison
Associate Editor: Siobhan Campbell
Production Manager: Christine Johnston
Design: Andy Chapman
Illustrator: Hardlines
Illustration Manager: Merlyn Harvey

Ultrasound Imaging for Rehabilitation of the Lumbopelvic Region

A Clinical Approach

Jackie L. Whittaker BScPT, FCAMT, CGIMS, CAFCI

Physiotherapist, Whittaker Physiotherapy Consulting, White Rock, B.C., Canada

Instructor, Orthopaedic Division of the Canadian Physiotherapy Association

Foreword by Maria Stokes PhD, MCSP

Professor of Neuromuscular Rehabilitation, School of Health Professions and Rehabilitation Sciences, University of Southampton, Southampton, UK

Formerly Director of Research and Development, Institute of Complex Neuro-disability, Royal Hospital for Neuro-disability, London, UK

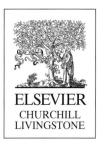

ELSEVIER
CHURCHILL
LIVINGSTONE

Edinburgh   London   New York   Oxford   Philadelphia   St Louis   Sydney   Toronto   2007

ELSEVIER
CHURCHILL
LIVINGSTONE

An imprint of Elsevier Limited

First published 2007

© 2007, Elsevier Ltd

ISBN-10: 0 443 06856 9
ISBN-13: 978 0 443 06856 0

British Library Cataloguing in Publication Data
A catalogue record for this book is available from the British Library.

Library of Congress Cataloging in Publication Data
A catalog record for this book is available from the Library of Congress.

Note
Neither the Publisher nor the Authors assume any responsibility for any loss or injury and/or damage to persons or property arising out of or related to any use of the material contained in this book. It is the responsibility of the treating practitioner, relying on independent expertise and knowledge of the patient, to determine the best treatment and method of application for the patient.

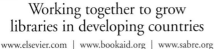

Working together to grow
libraries in developing countries

www.elsevier.com | www.bookaid.org | www.sabre.org

ELSEVIER   BOOK AID International   Sabre Foundation

your source for books,
journals and multimedia
in the health sciences

www.elsevierhealth.com

Printed in China

Contents

Foreword

Ultrasound imaging (USI) is probably most well known for examining the developing foetus, and is used as a diagnostic and guiding tool in many branches of medicine. Its potential use in rehabilitation was first indicated in the late 1960s and then highlighted by research on quadriceps muscle wasting in the 1980s. The technique has since been shown to provide an accurate, reliable, non-invasive means of evaluating muscles in terms of their size, shape and architecture, and the effects of different pathologies and interventions have been documented. Muscle size is related to the force it exerts, giving an indirect measure of strength, although the closeness of this relationship varies between muscles.

Muscles studied to date include: the lumbar multifidus, antero-lateral abdominal, posterior cervical spine, pelvic floor and anterior tibial muscles, as well as gastrocnemius, masseter, trapezius and the diaphragm. Much of the exploratory work has provided normal reference ranges and established the validity and reliability of the technique as a research tool.

Advances over the past decade in understanding the mechanisms of motor control and neuromusclar dysfunction, particularly of the stabilising muscles around joint complexes, prompted clinical interest in USI, as it provides a non-invasive means of detecting activity of deep muscles. Clinical application has been mainly for biofeedback to provide visual evidence of contraction to aid rehabilitation. There is particular interest in imaging the antero-lateral abdominal and multifidus muscles in the lumbopelvic region in association with low back pain, while pelvic floor imaging is a promising adjunct to the management of urinary incontinence in women's health.

For adoption of USI into routine physical therapy practice to be successful, guidelines and formal training are needed, using standardised protocols. A Symposium in San Antonio, Texas, in May

2006 was set up to develop practice guidelines and an international collaborative research agenda. Leading researchers in the field agreed definitions and guidance on imaging the abdominal, pelvic and posterior paraspinal muscles. The term Rehabilitative Ultrasound Imaging (RUSI) was formed and a consensus statement defined it as '. . . *a procedure used by physical therapists to evaluate muscle and related soft-tissue morphology and behavior during physical tasks . . . This includes providing feedback to the patient and physical therapist to improve clinical outcomes.*' This event was an important turning point in the field, clearly establishing RUSI as a recognised part of physical therapy practice. The outcomes of the Symposium are due to appear in a special issue of the *Journal of Orthopaedic and Sports Physical Therapy* in 2007, and the abstracts are already available (Teyhen 2006).

The definition of RUSI distinguishes it clearly from diagnostic musculoskeletal USI, which assesses ligament, tendon and muscle injuries, requiring different skills and training. In North America, physical therapists are not permitted to use USI for diagnosis of musculoskeletal conditions, while in other locations, such as the UK, therapists can undertake specific training. Since RUSI requires knowledge of functional anatomy of the muscular system and is integral to physical management of patients, by aiding evaluation and treatment, it does not encroach on the work of established imaging disciplines. Respecting professional boundaries and avoiding confusion with diagnostic musculoskeletal imaging will help ensure the acceptance by other disciplines of RUSI becoming part of routine physical therapy practice.

This book is the first practical guide on RUSI and is urgently needed. It outlines the background physics and then focuses on imaging the muscles of the lumbopelvic region and the bladder. Its author, Jackie Whittaker, is a highly skilled clinician and educator, who integrates research with clinical application, acknowledging throughout the book that much of the theoretical basis of existing clinical approaches requires further evidence. Some of the practical details of RUSI have yet to be standardised to minimise inconsistencies between groups and countries, and aligned as far as possible with established sonography practice. The author is one of the RUSI Symposium delegates still developing the international practice guidelines, so is well placed to offer her expertise. This informative, clearly presented reference guide provides an excellent introduction to RUSI and should prove to be a valuable resource to support training programmes.

Maria Stokes PhD MCSP
Professor of Neuromuscular Rehabilitation
University of Southampton, UK

REFERENCE

Teyhen D 2006 Rehabilitative Ultrasound Imaging Symposium, San Antonio, Texas, May 2006 Journal of Orthopaedic & Sports Physical Therapy 36(8):A1–A17

Preface

In the last decade there has been considerable growth in the knowledge base that serves as the foundation for neuromusculoskeletal rehabilitation. In particular, extensive focus has been placed upon identifying the neuromuscular mechanisms consistent with health, and the specific alterations that underlie dysfunction, such as low-back and pelvic girdle pain. Alongside this work, a valuable tool, **ultrasound imaging**, has emerged to assist clinicians in the detection and treatment of these neuromuscular or motor control impairments. However, what has not materialized are the resources needed to educate rehabilitation professionals in its use and clinical application.

When I began using ultrasound imaging to augment the management of patients with lumbopelvic dysfunction (lumbopelvic pain with associated continence and respiratory dysfunction), resources (both in the form of literature and clinical expertise) were limited. They consisted of a small section in a text, several research papers containing vague descriptions of methodology, and a handful of clinicians spread out around the globe. Over the last five years the popularity of the tool has increased, as has the scientific literature employing it. However, the information remains dispersed and disconnected. The aim of this text is to draw together published evidence with practical expertise, and present the first comprehensive resource for the rehabilitation clinician interested in integrating ultrasound imaging into their practice.

From a historical perspective, investigation into the nature and possible uses of ultrasound waves began in the 1920s, with initial medical applications introduced in the late 1930s. The focus of this early work centred on heating tissue for therapeutic purposes, with diagnostic applications following in the 1950s. Since that time, diagnostic imaging has been primarily concerned with traditional radiological goals, which consider morphological characteristics and structural integrity. However, as the technology has been embraced as a safe, portable, objective and relatively inexpensive means of examination, the ingenuity and diversity of applications has exploded.

Ultrasound imaging related to musculoskeletal rehabilitation has been ongoing since the 1980s. Current applications include assessment of muscle morphology (length, depth, diameter, cross-sectional area, volume), architectural changes in muscles and associated structures (fascia and organs such as the bladder) with muscle contraction, integrity of fascia, and motion of neurological tissue. Clinically, ultrasound imaging is a powerful tool as its dynamic, real-time nature allows clinicians to gather previously unavailable information about the status of the myofascial system, provide unparalleled visual feedback to their patients, and monitor the effectiveness of their treatment more objectively. Furthermore, it serves to refine the accuracy of a clinician's palpatory and observational skills in detecting subtle contractions in muscles that are deep and difficult to directly access.

Ultrasound imaging and in particular, real-time ultrasound imaging (the rapid sequential display of ultrasound images resulting in a moving presentation) is highly operator dependent. Clinicians embarking upon a journey to incorporate it into their daily practice require theoretical knowledge, as well as practical skill. Specifically, ultrasound imaging presents three major challenges:

- *Image generation* – the ability to use ultrasound technology to generate an image of the structure(s) of interest.
- *Image recognition* – the ability to orientate to the plane and anatomical structure(s) seen within the two-dimensional image.
- *Image interpretation* – the ability to interpret the still and dynamic images that are generated.

This text addresses these issues as they pertain to rehabilitation of neuromuscular dysfunction in the lumbopelvic region. It begins with a review of the basic principles of sound wave propagation, as well as a discussion of instrumentation, prudent use and safety topics (Chapter 1). Chapter 2 outlines, in a step-by-step fashion, the practicalities involved in generating images of the deep muscles and structures (fascia) that play a role in respiration, continence and postural control of the lumbopelvic region. This is followed by an in-depth discussion of the fundamentals of interpretation from both a qualitative (Chapter 3) and quantitative perspective (Chapter 4). The last chapter provides clinical guidance for the use of real-time ultrasound in the treatment of individuals with lumbopelvic dysfunction and addresses the value that it holds for both the therapist and the patient. The text concludes with appendices containing resources that facilitate the implementation of the technology into clinical practice, guidelines for accreditation, and a case study that provides a practical illustration of the way in which ultrasound imaging can enhance patient management. For those new to the technology it is critical to realize that it takes time to accumulate the knowledge, and perfect the skills, required for accurate interpretation and measurement. Hence the information contained here is only a beginning.

Although ultrasound imaging is currently used both in clinical and research settings, I believe that its full significance with regard to the rehabilitation process has yet to be revealed. The goal of this text is to give a comprehensive description of the current applications of ultrasound imaging in the rehabilitation of neuromusculoskeletal dysfunction in the lumbopelvic region based upon published evidence and clinical expertise. In doing so it is my hope to inspire further debate and research, as well as facilitate a greater understanding of the complementary role that ultrasound imaging can play in the rehabilitation of this region.

JW
White Rock, Canada
2007

Acknowledgements

As this text is a blending of the clinical and scientific worlds, I would like to begin by acknowledging two very important groups of people. First, the many individuals who have provided the evidence base for the material presented in this text. I convey my thanks, and express a sincere appreciation for their foresight, writings and outstanding work. Secondly, I extend enormous gratitude to the individuals and therapists who have shaped the clinical environments that I have had the opportunity to be a part of in the last thirteen years, as well as the students and patients who have served as a perpetual impetus for growth.

I wish to thank the production team from Elsevier (Heidi Harrison, Siobhan Campbell, and Christine Johnston) for their enthusiasm and support during this daunting task, as well as extend my gratitude to Ashley Smith and Alison McGrath. Ashley for his photographic skills (not to mention introducing me to that first ultrasound unit), and Alison both for her friendship, as well as for agreeing to serve as a model for the images in the text (not bad for a mom of two very robust little boys).

My journey into ultrasound imaging has been facilitated by Richard Boothroyd, Donna Ferri and Paul Muller of Biosound Esaote Inc. I pass on my deepest appreciation and thanks for their steadfast support over the last five years.

There is a quote from Isaac Newton which states *"If I have seen further it is by standing on the shoulders of giants"*. When it comes to the use of ultrasound imaging by physiotherapists these giants include Dr. Maria Stokes. I have been very fortunate to have had the opportunity to make her acquaintance, and am very honoured that she has agreed to write the foreword for this text.

There are countless individuals who have contributed to my professional growth and ultimately this project. In particular I would like to acknowledge my manual therapy mentors, Jim Meadows, and Erl Pettman, as well as Maureen Mooney. I have been blessed to have mentors that have turned into colleagues and in Maureen's case a wonderful friend. I need to acknowledge a genuine appreciation for colleagues Anne-Marie Fafard, Pat Fonstad, Linda-Joy Lee, Laurie McLaughlin, Tyla Schlender, Claire Small, Dan Siverston, Britt Stuge, as well as Deydre Teyhen. You have each contributed in your own special way whether it was through editorial comments, tenacious inquiry, enduring support or, through example. Diane Lee it is difficult to know what to write. You have been a steady influence, thank you for all that you have shared, and the path of discovery it has opened for me.

During this project I have been very fortunate to have had friends (many already mentioned) who continued to offer encouragement as well as places of solitude where I could work, and although I am not sure mention here does this support the justice that it deserves, I convey my deepest appreciation.

Finally, the last thanks is to OZ for their unconditional love, not to mention perseverance, to wait for that walk just another paragraph or two!!

'The voyage of discovery is not in seeking new landscapes but in having new eyes.'

MARCEL PROUST

1 Imaging principles and instrumentation

The initial challenges associated with real-time ultrasound imaging (RTUS) involve image generation and recognition. In addition to sound anatomical knowledge, these abilities require a fundamental understanding of the principles of sound wave propagation and ultrasound instrumentation. This chapter will review basic information on these topics, including the effect of varying frequencies and tissue boundaries on sound wave propagation, image resolution and artefacts, as well as discuss the generic characteristics of the technology, which are critical for orientating and manipulating the generated image (so-called 'knobology'). Issues related to safe and prudent use of ultrasound imaging (USI) by rehabilitation professionals will also be presented. The reader is encouraged to refer to the numerous articles and texts that exist for further discussion on the technical aspects presented here (Stokes et al 1997, Van Holsbeeck & Introcas 2001, Kremkau 2002).

PRINCIPLES OF SOUND WAVE PROPAGATION

The principles underlying the nature, generation and propagation of ultrasound waves are consistent across therapeutic and diagnostic applications. The principal difference between the two lies in the frequency and intensity of the sound wave used, as well as the fact that in diagnostic applications the reflections (echoes) of the sound waves are captured and used to generate an image.

Ultrasound waves are generated by short electrical impulses that are passed across crystalline structures referred to as 'transducers'. The electrical impulses vibrate the transducer and are correspondingly converted into very high frequency (ultra) sound waves. This phenomenon of converting electrical signals into ultrasonic sound waves is termed a 'reverse piezoelectric effect'. Although the number

1

and orientation of the crystalline structures can vary depending on the specific probe, the basic principle is consistent. A feature distinct to imaging units is that the transducer is also capable of collecting reflected sound waves and converting them back into an electrical signal (piezoelectric effect), which can then be used to create a digital image. Specifically, imaging units generate pulses of ultrasound waves that are sent into the body, where they produce reflections (echoes) at organ boundaries and within tissues. The echoes return to the transducer and then are processed and displayed as visible dots (pixels). The brightness of a pixel depends upon echo strength, which in turn is determined by the location and specific characteristics of the echo-generating structure. The position or plot of a pixel is established by considering the direction of an ultrasound wave when it entered the body, the length of time it takes for the echo to return to the transducer, and the speed at which sound can travel through soft tissue (Kremkau 2002). To competently generate and interpret ultrasound images one must understand the nature of the echo, hence properties of sound wave propagation.

Ultrasound is a delineation given to sound waves with a frequency greater than what can be perceived by the human auditory system (>20,000 Hz). Although these waves are unique they propagate according to principles that apply to all sound waves. If one was to bang on a drum, a sound wave would be created. How far the sound could be heard and whether an echo was produced would depend on how the drum was hit, the properties of the medium that the sound had to travel through and the number, shape and properties of the objects that it encountered. Similar to the sound wave produced by a drum, ultrasound waves travel through some media better than others, and can virtually bounce off of and be absorbed by anything. These behaviours can be summarized by three basic principles: penetration, attenuation and reflection.

Penetration

Penetration refers to the ability of sound to travel. In the context of ultrasound, penetration is influenced by the intensity (strength or 'loudness') of an ultrasound beam, as well as the frequency and speed of the sound waves within the beam. The intensity of an ultrasound beam is defined as the rate at which energy is delivered per unit area. It is determined by the total power output of the probe (watts, W) divided by its area (cm^2), and is expressed in units of milliwatts per square centimetre (mW/cm^2). As the intensity of a sound beam increases so does the strength of the echo that it has the potential to produce, and the depth it can penetrate. In addition to its influence on echo strength and penetration intensity is the key to heat production, and as a general rule the greater the intensity the greater the associated increase in tissue temperature. Diagnostic ultrasound applications employ significantly lower (0.005–0.03 W/cm^2) intensities than therapeutic applications (0.5–3 W/cm^2) and result in negligible increases in tissue temperature.

Frequency is defined as the number of oscillations that a wave undergoes in one second and is expressed in hertz (Hz): 1 Hz = 1 oscillation or cycle per second; 1 kilohertz (kHz) = 1000 oscillations per second; 1 megahertz (MHz) = 1 million oscillations per second (Michlovitz 1990). The higher the frequency of sound the less the emerging wave will diverge. Consequently, ultrasound waves are very cohesive (similar to a light beam leaving a laser pointer) and can be used to selectively expose a limited target area. The most common frequencies employed with ultrasound imaging are 3.5–10 MHz. The frequency of an ultrasound wave is determined in the construction of a probe, with most capable of generating two distinct frequencies (e.g. 3.5–5.0 MHz or 7.5–10.0 MHz). As a general rule the lower the frequency of a sound wave the deeper it will penetrate.

The speed at which an ultrasound wave travels is determined by the compressibility (molecular structure) or 'hardness' of the medium it is traversing (Kremkau 2002). The more rigid or 'hard' the material the faster sound travels through it. The average speed at which sound travels through soft tissue is 1540 metres per second (m/s) (Michlovitz 1990). This is very close to the velocity that it would travel through water (1485–1526 m/s). Fat is less stiff than most soft tissue, hence sound traverses it slightly slower (1460 m/s). Muscle and bone are more stiff and consequently, sound can propagate faster (1585 m/s and 4080 m/s respectively) (Stokes et al 1997). As the speed of sound in soft tissue is relatively constant, ultrasound imaging units are calibrated to assume that sound travels through all tissues at 1540 m/s.

Attenuation

As an ultrasound wave traverses the distance between the transducer and the target tissue it will be reflected and absorbed at boundaries between media of dissimilar acoustic properties. Hence the energy within the sound wave decreases as it penetrates until it is completely dispersed. This phenomenon, referred to as attenuation, is fundamental to image generation.

Attenuation is a result of reflection, scattering and absorption. When sound waves hit a tissue interface they break up or fracture. These fractions are delineated by whether they are reflected back to where they came from, scattered in another direction or absorbed.

If the fractured portion of sound wave is deflected as a result of striking the tissue interface then the term scattering or reflection is used. If the energy of the fractured portion of the sound wave is transferred to the surrounding tissue (in the form of heat), it is referred to as absorption. It is interesting to note that attenuation occurs primarily (80%) through absorption, and only a small portion of the original sound wave is ever reflected or scattered.

The practical implication of attenuation is that it limits penetration and consequently the depth of images that can be generated (Kremkau 2002). Attenuation and frequency have a direct relationship. The higher the frequency of an ultrasound wave (10 MHz) the greater the attenuation and the more shallow its penetration. Conversely, the greater the attenuation, the more echo (reflection) created and the better the resolution of the ultrasound image (**Fig. 1.1**). Consequently, the choice of frequency used for an imaging application will be dependent upon the depth of the region or structures of interest. Higher frequencies (7.5–10 MHz) are more valuable for examining superficial structures (superficial muscles, ligaments and tendons), and lower frequencies (3.5–5 MHz) for deeper structures (deeper muscles, the bladder and the contents of the abdominal/pelvic cavities). As a general rule the highest-frequency transducer which can image an area of interest should be used.

Reflection

Ultrasound technology is useful as an imaging tool due to the fact that sound waves are reflected at the border of, and within, heterogeneous media. Specifically, it is the reflections of the sound waves that produce the pattern of echoes that are then deciphered to generate an image. The pattern of reflected sound waves is dependent

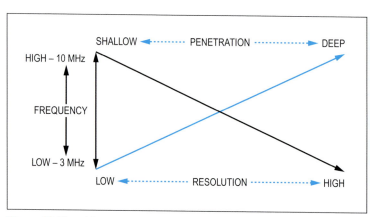

Figure 1.1 Pictorial representation of the relationship between image resolution, frequency and penetration of ultrasound waves.

upon the size of the reflecting medium, the roughness of its surface, the incident angle of the sound wave when it encountered the medium, and the difference in impedance of the two media that create the interface (Kremkau 2002). The more irregular the surface, the greater the difference in impedance, and the more perpendicular a sound wave encounters the interface, the greater the proportion of the deflection that will be reflected back to the transducer versus that which is lost to scattering or absorption.

The impedance of a medium is equal to its density multiplied by the speed at which ultrasound can propagate through it. Impedance increases if either the density or the propagation speed of the medium increase. The greater the difference in impedance between two media the greater the intensity of the echo generated at their interface and the brighter (more white) the interface is represented in the ensuing ultrasound image. If there is no difference in impedance between two media, no echo will be generated and nothing will be seen on the ultrasound screen. Alternatively, if there is a very large discrepancy in impedance between two media, such as air and soft tissue, there is total reflection of the sound wave (hence the need for a coupling medium such as gel or water) (Kremkau 2002). Throughout this text, the images generated are ones in which the tissue interfaces are quite obvious; however, the operator will need to differentiate between bone, muscle, fascia, fluid, fat and gas.

Bone is unique in that its density is so great it attenuates (absorbs/reflects) 100% of the sound that reaches it. The practical implications of this are that bone produces a substantial reflection (hyperechoic) which results in its surface appearing as a very bright white border within an ultrasound image (**Fig. 1.2a**). The echo strength of the border is further enhanced due to the significant difference in impedance between bone and muscle (Stokes et al 1997). A further consideration is that bone prevents the transmission of sound to structures that are deep to, distal, or on the other side of it. Thus, the area distal to bone within an ultrasound image is in a 'shadow', appears black, and contains no useful information. Clinically, it is important to consider that bone can impede the view of deeper structures (**Fig. 1.2b**); however, as it is stationary and easy to identify, it can also serve as a useful landmark.

The appearance of muscle within an ultrasound image can vary depending on its orientation, architecture, morphology and anatomical location. Generally healthy muscle contains a large degree of blood (hypoechoic), and the fascia that encapsulates and separates it from other layers or structures is less vascular and quite dense (hyperechoic). Consequently, muscle layers appear darker with fewer shades of grey and the encapsulating fascia appears quite white. Some regions such as the lateral abdominal wall are more dramatic examples of this delineation (**Fig. 1.3a**). Muscle that has

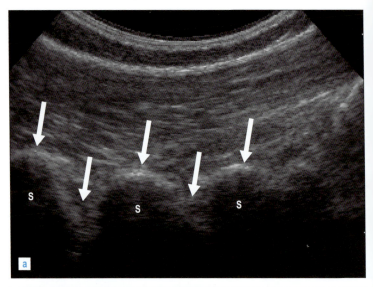

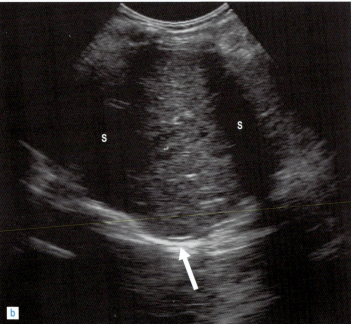

Figure 1.2 a. A sagittal ultrasound image of the lumbar vertebral column. Note the brightness of the muscle–bone interface (arrows) as well as the shadow (s) that exists deep to it. **b.** An ultrasound image of the diaphragm (arrow) taken through the rib cage. Note the shadows (s) produced by the ribs as they interfere with the propagation of the sound wave.

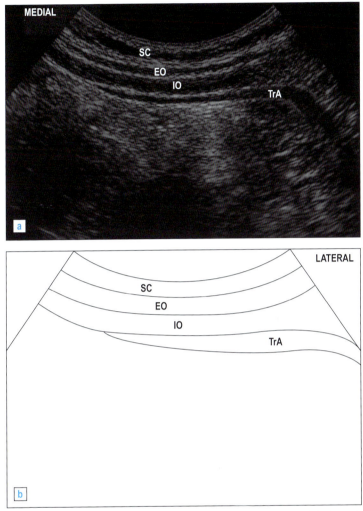

Figure 1.3 a. An ultrasound image of the muscle and fascia layers of the lateral abdominal wall. Note that the muscle layers are darker (hypoechoic), while the intervening fascia is brighter (hyperechoic). **b.** Labelled outline.
SC = subcutaneous tissue, EO = external oblique, IO = internal oblique.
TrA = transversus abdominis.

fatty fibrous tissue infiltration will have greater echogenicity and appear whiter. This is commonly seen with atrophy (Strobel et al 2005) as well as in older individuals (Stokes et al 2005).

The appearance of fluid (urine/blood) within an ultrasound image is distinctive. It is a medium that provides little impedance, causes minimal attenuation (absorption/reflection/scatter) and excels in transmitting sound waves. As a hypoechoic medium, fluid appears black within an ultrasound image (**Fig. 1.4a, b**) and facilitates the transmission of sound to structures that lie deep to, distal, or on

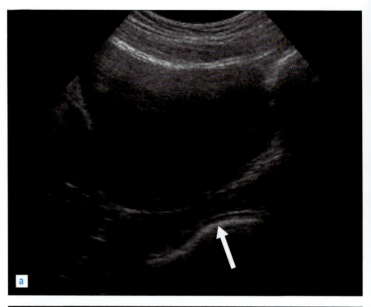

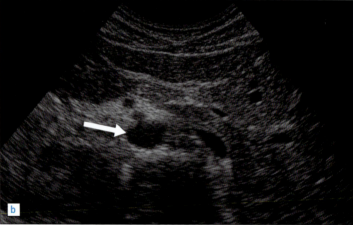

Figure 1.4 a. An ultrasound image of the bladder. Note both the hypoechoic nature (black) of the urine and how the fluid serves as an acoustic window allowing for visualization of the vaginal wall (arrow). **b.** An ultrasound image of the aorta (arrow). Again note the hypoechoic nature of the fluid which in this case is blood.

the other side of it. Consequently, it can be used as an 'acoustic window' allowing for views of deeper structures. A clinical example of this is a moderately full bladder serving as an acoustic window to view the vaginal wall (**Fig. 1.4a**).

Although image properties are largely dependent upon the difference in impedance between media, and the composition of the target tissue, it is important to recognize the influence of structures positioned along the path of the propagating sound wave between the transducer and the target tissue. For instance, abdominal gas, an increased subcutaneous fat layer, or muscle–fat combinations decrease the clarity of an image due to the scattering effect that fat and gas have on a sound wave (**Fig. 1.5a, b**). The effect of these media may partially obliterate the echo and lead to difficulties with interpretation and visualization of deeper structures (Haberkorn et al 1993).

Finally, it is important to remember that an ultrasound unit generates images based upon several assumptions: sound travels in

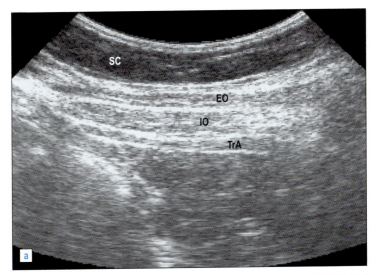

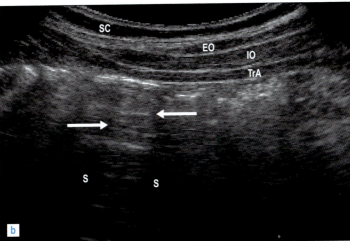

Figure 1.5 a. An ultrasound image of the lateral abdominal wall demonstrating the scattering effect of subcutaneous fat. Note the grainy appearance of the image, as well as the brightness depicted in the muscle layers. **b.** The appearance of the lateral abdominal wall without the scattering effect of adipose tissue. Note however the abdominal gas (arrows) and resulting shadows (s). SC = subcutaneous, EO = external oblique, IO = internal oblique, TrA = transversus abdominis.

straight lines; echoes only originate from objects located in the two dimensions of the sound beam; the amplitude of the echo is directly related to the reflecting or scattering properties of distant objects; and the speed at which sound travels through all tissues is 1540 m/s. If any of these assumptions is violated then incorrect representations of anatomy can occur (Kremkau 2002).

Artefact

Artefact refers to anything that is an incorrect representation of the anatomy (Kremkau 2002). Artefacts can be both helpful and a hindrance. They are produced by improper equipment operation, imaging technique, the physics of ultrasound or a violation of one of the multiple assumptions incorporated into the design of the ultrasound imaging instrument. They can be summarized as situations that result in structures that are either not real, missing, improperly located or of improper brightness, shape or size. Kremkau (2002) describes sixteen different artefacts; however, this text will only consider the two that will have the greatest impact on its readers: shadowing and enhancement.

Shadowing refers to a reduction in the sound wave echo from structures that lie behind a strongly reflecting or attenuating structure such as bone. Simply put, the ultrasound waves hit something that blocks their path and everything behind the blocking structure appears black as if they were within an 'acoustic shadow' (**Fig. 1.6a, b**). A shadow can also occur as a sound beam is refracted (bent) from its original path as it passes close to a large curved fluid-filled structure (e.g. bladder) (**Fig. 1.7a, b**). When this occurs the shadow is referred to as an 'edge artefact' or 'edge shadow', as it is seen to project from the edges of the curved structure.

The opposite of shadowing occurs when ultrasound waves encounter a structure that does little to reflect or absorb it, such as a fluid-filled cavity (e.g. bladder). This is referred to as enhancement, and it is defined as the strengthening of the echo distal to a weakly attenuating structure. Basically, the tissues on the far side of the transmitting structure appear more brightly than they should, as they are being exposed with a less attenuated beam (**Fig. 1.8a, b**).

INSTRUMENTATION

A typical medical ultrasound imaging device is a pulsed-echo (generates a series of short ultrasound waves at regular intervals) instrument consisting of two components: a transducer assembly or

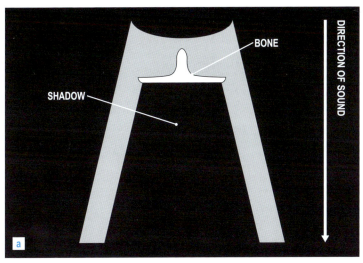

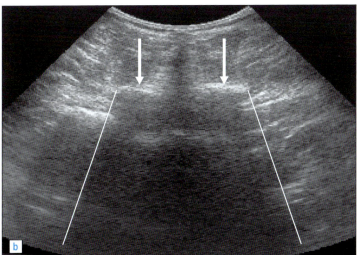

Figure 1.6 Acoustic shadowing. **a.** A depiction of how an acoustic shadow forms behind a strongly attenuating structure such as bone (adapted from Wiss 2002). **b.** An ultrasound image demonstrating acoustic shadowing (the outlined dark region) caused by the articular processes of a vertebra (arrows).

probe, and an imaging system. The transducer assembly is the component responsible for generating ultrasound waves, as well as where the ultrasound echoes returning from the tissues are received and converted into an electrical signal. Probes have individual characteristics dependent upon their design, and these along with their clinical implications will be considered below. The imaging system is the component of the technology that receives the electrical signal representing the echo from the transducer, and processes it so that it can be displayed as a digital image.

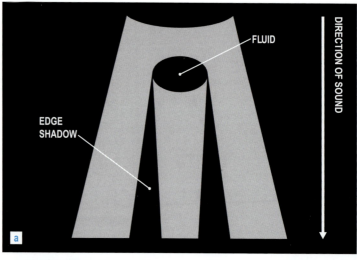

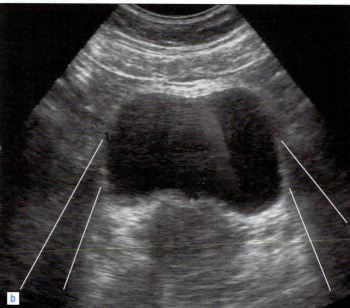

Figure 1.7 Edge shadowing. **a.** A depiction of an edge shadow produced when a sound wave is refracted around the edges of a fluid filled structure (adapted from Wiss 2002). **b.** An ultrasound image demonstrating edge shadowing (the dark outlined regions) caused by the bladder.

Imaging system

Medical ultrasound imaging systems contain four generic components (**Fig. 1.9**); the beam former, signal processor, image processor and display. The beam former is responsible for generating the

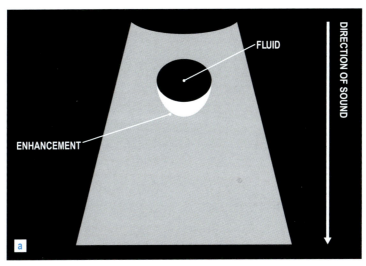

FLUID

DIRECTION OF SOUND

ENHANCEMENT

a

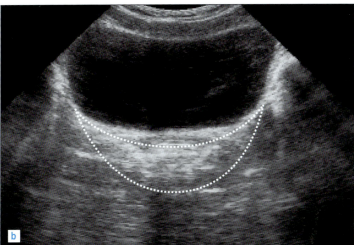

b

Figure 1.8 Enhancement. **a.** A depiction of the enhancement of a region deep to a fluid-filled structure. Enhancement occurs as the fluid-filled structure results in less attenuation of the propagating sound wave (adapted from Wiss 2002). **b.** An ultrasound image demonstrating enhancement (outlined crescent shape) of the midline pelvic floor structures deep to the bladder (the transmitting structure).

electrical impulses that drive the transducer, as well as for amplifying and digitalizing the electrical signal returning from the transducer that represents the ultrasound echo. After the electrical signal has been amplified and digitized by the beam former it is transferred onto the signal processor, where it is filtered and compressed before being sent on to the image processor. Finally, the image processor converts the digitized, filtered and compressed echo data into visual images and then presents them on the instrument's display (Kremkau 2002).

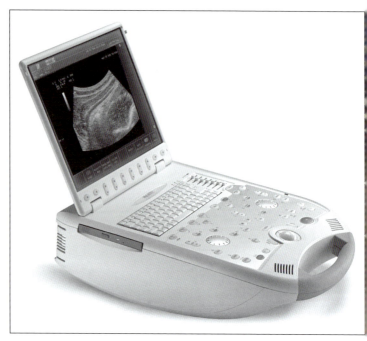

Figure 1.9 A typical medical ultrasound imaging system, MyLab 30 model – Biosound Esaote Inc., Indianapolis, Indiana, USA (reproduced with permission).

Transducer assembly

A transducer is a device that converts one form of energy to another. An ultrasound transducer is a device that converts electrical energy into ultrasound energy and vice versa. Ultrasound transducers (also referred to as elements or crystals), commonly a ceramic formulation of lead zirconate titanate, are piezoelectric elements that produce voltage when deformed by an applied pressure such as a sound wave (Kremkau 2002). The transducer elements, which are most commonly rectangular in shape, along with their associated casing and dampening material are referred to as the transducer assembly or probe. The arrangement and the operating frequency of the elements, as well as the width of the field of view (in metric) produced are all taken into consideration when describing a probe.

The arrangement, or array, of the elements within a probe can be linear or curved (also referred to as convex or sector). Both have distinct footprints and fields of view (**Fig. 1.10c, Fig. 1.11c**). A linear array probe typically consists of eighty, or more, small rectangular crystal elements mounted side by side to form a single strip. By triggering the elements sequentially, a rectangular ultrasound image is built up from many vertical, parallel scan lines with

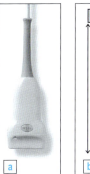
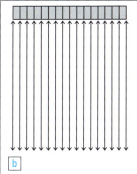
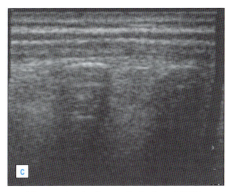

Figure 1.10 a. A linear array probe (7.5-10 MHz Biosound Esaote Inc., Indianapolis, Indiana, USA) (reproduced with permission). **b.** A pictorial representation of the transducer elements (grey squares) and their vertical, parallel scan lines (Kremkau 2002). **c.** An ultrasound image generated using a 7.5-10 MHz linear array probe. Note the linear footprint and the rectangular nature of the image.

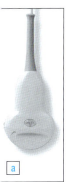
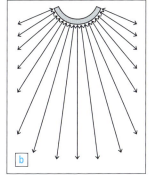
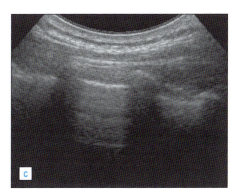

Figure 1.11 a. A curved or convex array probe (3.5-5 MHz Biosound Esaote Inc, Indianapolis, Indiana, USA) (reproduced with permission). **b.** A pictorial representation of the transducer array and the diverging scan lines of a curved or convex array probe (Kremkau 2002). **c.** An ultrasound image identical to Fig. 1.10C generated using a 3.5-5 MHz curved or convex array probe. Note the curved footprint and the pie or sector nature of the image.

a width that approximates the length of the array (Kremkau 2002). The advantage of a linear array is its wide near field, which is appropriate for imaging small superficial structures (**Fig. 1.10a, b, c**). Curved array technology is similar, except that the crystal elements are formed into a curve, rather than a straight line, which results in a diverging (pie or sector shaped) ultrasound image. The advantages of a curved array is its wide far field, coupled with a small 'footprint' which is suitable for imaging deep abdominal structures (**Fig. 1.11a, b, c**).

The frequency of a probe is predetermined by the thickness of the elements (the thicker the elements the lower the frequency) and the propagation speed of the transducer material. A typical transducer produces a range of frequencies around a maximal frequency which is referred to as the 'operating' or 'resonance' frequency. It is commonplace that a probe may have two distinct operating frequencies (e.g. 3.5 or 5.0 MHz vs. 7.5 or 10.0 MHz) and both are used to identify the probe. The majority of the ultrasound images found within this text have been generated with a 3.5-5 MHz curvilinear array probe with a 40 mm width.

EQUIPMENT CONTROLS

Ultrasound imaging units have a variety of controls. These can be divided into output and input functions. Output functions refer to controls that modulate how the ultrasound wave is generated, while input functions are related to reception, processing and display of the ultrasound echoes. Output controls (namely power) affect the degree of ultrasound exposure that the patient will experience, while input controls do not. The ultrasound operator requires a basic understanding of these functions so that they will be able to balance ultrasound exposure against the intensity required to adequately image a structure, as well as how to manipulate the ultrasound image to bring attention to the aspects of the image that are of interest. The major output function is power, while input functions include image depth, gain (total, near and far), brightness and contrast.

Power

The output power control (commonly labelled output, power, output power, transmit, damping or sensitivity) governs the amplitude of ultrasound pulses and (as the area of the transducer is constant) the intensity of the ultrasound beam. Increasing the output power increases the quantity of sound that is sent into the body. As the amount of sound sent into the body increases so does the strength of the echoes that it generates, and the amount of sound that is attenuated as heat. Hence, the output power control should be manipulated such that an adequate image of the structure of interest is generated with a minimal amount of ultrasound exposure (see ALARA principle under 'safety guidelines' below). This is of greatest importance in applications that involve exposure of tissues that are at risk of increasing in temperature, such as foetal bone (see 'thermal effects' below).

Image depth

The depth and size of the field of view of the image on display can be increased or decreased by manipulating the image depth controls on the ultrasound unit (**Fig. 1.12a, b**). Ultimately, the upper and lower limits of these selections depend upon the frequency of a probe; however, there is some flexibility, allowing attention to be focused towards either superficial or deeper structures. The applications in this text deal primarily with relatively superficial structures (abdominal wall, lumbar multifidus), hence the depth control setting

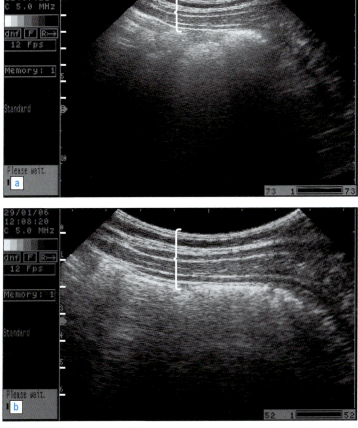

Figure 1.12 Demonstration of depth control. **a.** A transverse image of the lateral abdominal wall in which the field of view and depth have been maximized allowing for exposure of deeper structures. **b.** An identical image to **A**; however, the field of view and depth have been minimized, allowing for a closer inspection of the superficial structures (which in this case are the muscles of the lateral abdominal wall). Note that the hash marks on the left side of the display represent an equal distance (1 cm) in both images; what differs between the images is the scale.

will correspond. However, deeper settings will be employed in all applications involving imaging of the bladder (see Chapter 2).

Gain, brightness and contrast

Gain refers to the degree of amplification that the beam former imparts to the electrical signal (representing the echo) coming from the transducer. This degree of amplification can be modified in most units by manipulating the total, near or far gain controls. With too little gain weak echoes are not displayed, while with too much gain all echoes are revealed, saturation occurs, and differentiation between structures is made difficult (**Fig. 1.13a, b**). In normal situations in which the operator wants a uniform density throughout the image the total gain and depth gain controls should be set in their mid-range. However, for certain applications this may not be suitable. If the overall gain of the ultrasound image needs to be altered, the total gain control is manipulated. If the gain at a certain depth needs to be altered, the near (top half of the display) or far (bottom half of the display) gain controls can be utilized. Manipulation of the gain controls is often situation-specific and depends upon the preference of the operator. Generic guidelines with respect to the applications in this text will be outlined in the following chapters. In addition to the gain controls, all ultrasound imaging units have controls for manipulating the brightness and contrast of the display screen itself.

Modes of display

There are several options (modes) available for the display, or presentation of the echoes returning to the ultrasound transducer. The most common display modes encountered in rehabilitation applications are B (brightness, brilliance) and M (motion, movement).

'B' or brightness (brilliance) mode is the cross-sectional grey-scale image typically associated with ultrasound applications (**Fig. 1.14a**). B-mode images use dots of various degrees of brightness to represent the location and density of the structures located within the ultrasound beam. More specifically, the brightness of each dot is determined by the strength of the returning echo. The images displayed in B mode reflect information gathered from the entire length of the transducer and they allow the investigator to view the 'main event' and its impact on all structures within the field of view.

'M' or motion mode illustrates the motion of a structure by displaying its depth over time (**Fig. 1.14b**). Data are collected from

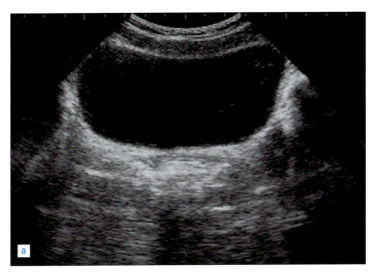

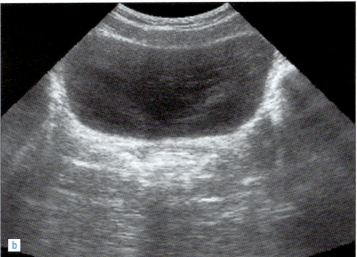

Figure 1.13 Demonstration of gain control. **a.** A transverse image of the bladder in which the total gain has been minimized. Note that the appearances of structures that generate weak echoes (such as the superior border of the bladder) are lost. **b.** An identical image to 'A' in which the gain control has been increased such that the structures with weaker echoes are now more visible.

the midpoint of a probe and is presented as a continuous image over time. The image has a tramline effect with the lines representing tissue boundaries. Stationary structures appear as a straight line, while moving ones will create a wave pattern in which frequency and excursion can be measured. M mode is typically used in cardiac applications; however, it may have a role to play in the assessment of the muscles of the lateral abdominal wall (Bunce et al 2002,

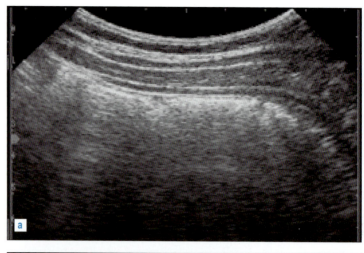

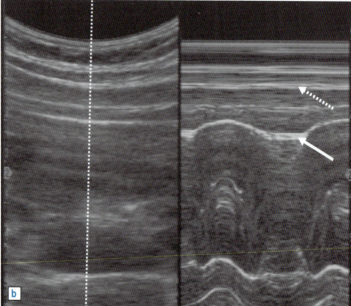

Figure 1.14 a. A typical B-mode image of the lateral abdominal wall. **b.** A split-screen image with B mode on the left and M mode on the right. The dotted line on the B-mode image represents the point from which the M-mode display data is being gathered. That is, the M-mode image represents the information from the dotted line displayed over time. Static structures are represented with straight lines (dotted arrow) and structures that move (in this case the transversus abdominis) are represented by curved lines (straight arrow).

2004). Typical ultrasound imaging units have the capability of both B and M-mode displays, as well as split-screen options (one side of the screen is in B mode, while the other is in M mode) (**Fig. 1.14b**). The images found in this text are all displayed in B mode.

SCOPE OF PRACTICE

The use of USI by a clinician is dictated by their specific profession and its scope of practice. For example, the scope of practice of physiotherapy generally refers to

the assessment and treatment of neuro-musculoskeletal and cardio-respiratory systems of the body by physical or mechanical means, for the purpose of maintenance or restoration of function, that has been impaired by injury or disease, for pain management and for the promotion of mobility and health . . .

(WCPT 1999)

This statement verifies that the rehabilitation of movement dysfunction and the neuromusculoskeletal system is within the scope of practice of the physiotherapy profession. It also confirms that a physiotherapist is qualified and allowed by his/her professional scope to establish a physical diagnosis and determine a client's movement potential, as well as to plan and implement physiotherapy programmes, using specialized knowledge, skills and tools for the prevention or treatment of movement dysfunction.

In the last decade there has been considerable growth in the knowledge base that is the foundation for neuromusculoskeletal rehabilitation. In particular, extensive focus has been placed upon identifying the neuromuscular mechanisms consistent with health, and the specific alterations that underlie dysfunction. From this work it has become evident that a primary impairment seen in chronic cervical, low-back and pelvic-girdle pain is one of altered neuromuscular control as opposed to decreased strength or functional capacity (Jull & Richardson 2000, Hodges & Moseley 2003, Falla et al 2004a, b, Richardson et al 2004, Cholewicki et al 2005, Stuge et al 2006a). Alongside the emerging evidence, clinical tools have materialized (namely USI) that aid physiotherapists and other rehabilitation professionals in the detection and treatment of this altered motor control (Hides et al 1995b, Stokes et al 1997).

USI has been established as a safe, cost-effective (as opposed to the alternative of magnetic resonance imaging) and accessible method for visualizing and measuring the deep muscles of the trunk (Bernstein et al 1991, Hides et al 1995a, Blaney et al 1999, Bunce et al 2002, Hodges et al 2003a). The value of USI to rehabilitation is that it allows for dynamic study (real-time images) of muscle groups as they contract. Consequently the complementary use of USI can enhance the clinical analysis of these muscles and has been advocated by various authors (Hides et al 1995b, Stokes et al 1997, Richardson et al 2004, Kermode 2004, Whittaker 2004a, b, Henry & Westervelt 2005). In addition to its safety and accessibility record it is imperative to note that USI has withstood scientific rigour and has been shown to be valid and reliable when applied in a thoughtful manner (Hides et al 1992, Blaney et al 1999, Schaer et al 1999, Bunce et al 2002, 2004, Coldron et al 2003, Ferreira et al 2004, Stokes et al 2005, Ainscough-Potts et al 2006).

USI should be viewed as a tool, in the same light as say, a stethoscope. A variety of health care professionals employ a stethoscope during their daily practice. Dependent on the information sought, their unique area of training and level of knowledge, the tool is used differently (Wiss 2002). The uses of USI by rehabilitation professionals may vary depending on jurisdiction, its specific licensing guidelines and professional regulation. In a report to the College of Physical Therapists of British Columbia, Canada (Whittaker 2004c) a generic definition regarding the use of USI by physiotherapists that encompasses current clinical practices has been proposed and includes 'applications that result in a physical diagnosis of the size or movement characteristics of muscles and/or nerves in relation to adjacent structures'. At present it is not universally within the scope of practice of physiotherapists to make a medical diagnosis of altered tissue morphology based on the interpretation of an imaging study.

In the current environment of evidence-based practice and fiscal accountability it is imperative that rehabilitation professionals be allowed access to the tools that optimize the effectiveness of their interventions and implement the growing knowledge base. It is important, however, that each profession determine how they can best use this tool to benefit their patients and rise to the challenge of defending their scope of practice if it is challenged. However, contiguous to this task is the responsibility associated with quality control, accreditation and development of policies to ensure the safe and appropriate use of the technology by the members of each profession. It is imperative that all rehabilitation professionals that employ USI are qualified to do so, are aware of their scope of practice and adhere to it.

SAFETY CONSIDERATIONS

The World Health Organization (WHO) has stated that 'the benefits of this imaging (ultrasound) modality far outweigh any presumed risks' (WHO 1982, 1989). Although the potential for harm does exist when human tissue is exposed to any energy it is important to appreciate that due to the extensive research and development that has taken place in the last 90 years, as well as the level of regulation that the technology has undergone, it has an exemplary safety record. Countless studies have been conducted and no known risks have been identified (Nyborg 2001, Kremkau 2002). Consequently, the discussion that follows is one based on theoretical prudence, ensuring that professionals who employ USI are aware of the basis for potential harm and use common sense in determining the suitability of the patient and the type of scan to perform.

Ultrasound waves produce mechanical vibration of the particles of a medium (tissue). This vibration is cyclical and allows for propagation of the ultrasound energy. In addition to this propagation the vibration can also produce localized forces and stresses within the medium. Hence when ultrasound is applied to human tissues a variety of events can occur. In general, these events or effects can be classified as either thermal or non-thermal, and are determined by characteristics of the ultrasound beam (intensity) and the size of the area and type of tissue exposed, as well as the length of the exposure.

Thermal effects

Thermal effects refer to the heating of the tissues that results from the attenuation of the ultrasound beam as it propagates through tissues. The potential for an increase in tissue temperature is present (and desirable in most therapeutic applications) with all uses of ultrasound; however, harm can result in circumstances where the rise is greater than 2°C. The extent of the temperature rise depends on the intensity (power) and frequency of the sound waves, as well as the perfusion of the exposed tissue. The higher the intensity or frequency and the poorer the perfusion of the region, the greater the temperature increase will be. As bone is the most efficient tissue for converting ultrasound energy to heat, theoretical consideration should always be taken when it is one of the tissues to be exposed, and more specifically, in obstetric applications where the ultrasound wave may impose on developing, poorly perfused, foetal skeletal tissue (Nyborg 2002). However, this being said, extreme experiments (during which guinea pig and rat foetal skeletal tissue was exposed to high-intensity ultrasound for up to 50 hours), have failed to demonstrate an increase in tissue temperature greater than 2°C, nor consequential abnormality development (Nyborg 2002).

In summary, the American Institute of Ultrasound in Medicine (AIUM 2000) concludes that with respect to heat:

- 'Excessive temperature increase can result in toxic effects in mammals'.

- 'For [ultrasound] exposure up to 50 hrs in duration, there have been no significant, adverse biological effects observed due to temperature increases less than or equal to 2°C above normal'.

- 'In general adult tissues are more tolerant of temperature increases than fetal and neonatal tissues'.

- 'For similar exposure conditions, the expected temperature increase in bone is significantly greater than in soft tissues. For this reason, conditions where an ultrasound impinges on ossifying fetal bone deserve special attention due to its close proximity to other developing tissues'.

Non-thermal effects

The most common non-thermal effect associated with ultrasound is cavitation. Cavitation refers to the production and behaviour of gas bubbles within a liquid. When ultrasound travels through a fluid it can generate tiny bubbles from the dissolved gases within the fluids that it encounters. The behaviour of these gas bubbles in response to the fluctuations in pressure associated with the ultrasound beam can be variable, and is influenced by factors such as the size of the cavity, and the nature of the immediate environment (Nyborg 2002). At one extreme, gas bubbles within a cavity or tissue may respond with small volume oscillations that are synchronized with the ultrasound wave (stable cavitation). At the other extreme, these bubbles may respond with large unsynchronized oscillations which lead them to slowly expand then suddenly collapse into a greatly reduced volume. This implosion can be quite violent, increase the pressure and temperature of the gaseous contents, and be damaging to the surrounding tissue (haemorrhaging etc.). The literature would suggest that the gas-filled adult lungs are the primary location susceptible to ultrasonic haemorrhaging (foetal lung tissue does not contain gas) as a result of cavitation. However, another consideration would be a situation in which an individual may have had a gaseous contrast agent injected and remnants make cavitation and tissue damage (e.g. capillary damage within muscle) more probable (Miller & Quddus 2000).

In summary, the American Institute of Ultrasound in Medicine (AIUM 2000) concludes that with respect to cavitation:

- 'Thus far, biologically significant, adverse, non-thermal effects (cavitation resulting in extravasation of blood cells) have only been identified with certainty for diagnostically relevant exposures in tissues that have well defined populations of stabilized gas bodies'.

- 'Furthermore, for diagnostically relevant exposures no independently confirmed biologically significant adverse non-thermal effects have been reported in mammalian tissues that do not contain well defined gas bodies'.

Prudent use

Although there are no confirmed biological effects on humans caused by exposure from present diagnostic ultrasound instruments, the possibility exists that such biological effects may be identified in the future (AIUM 2000, Kremkau 2002, Nyborg 2002). Thus USI should be used in a prudent manner, as outlined below, to provide therapeutic benefit. Moreover, it is important to consider that prudent use may relate to the lack of standardized training, rather than to inherent risks associated with the devices themselves. These issues, however, can ultimately be addressed through the introduction and enforcement of clinical standards of practice, the implementation of sound accreditation processes and regular (yearly) maintenance and calibration of the imaging devices (Hedrick 1995, Whittaker 2004c).

Based upon a review of the literature (Hedrick 1995, AIUM 2000, Kremkau 2002, Nyborg 2002) generic safety guidelines regarding prudent use and clinical standards for the application of USI by physiotherapists have been developed (Whittaker 2004c) and are presented here. Further reflection and discussion will be necessary in light of the emergence of future evidence.

Safety guidelines

USI and pregnancy:

In accordance with the recommendations by the NCRP (National Council for Radiation Protection and Measurements – USA) an exposure of less than five minutes is unlikely to result in an increase in temperature of greater that 2°C. Thus any imaging applications which will involve exposure to the foetus should be kept to duration of less than five minutes.

USI and the lungs/intestines:

In accordance with the NCRP a risk–benefit decision is important when imaging aerated lung tissue or intestine which contains significant gas bodies. Thus any imaging applications which involve exposure of these tissues should be kept to duration of less than five minutes.

Gaseous contrast media:

Diagnostic ultrasound should not be applied to individuals who have *recently* undergone the injection of gaseous contrast medium to the region that is to be imaged.

ALARA principle:

All rehabilitation professionals using USI in their practice should be aware of and employ the ALARA principle. ALARA is an acronym for 'As Low As Reasonably Achievable'. This principle suggests that USI should be used when indicated, in a way in which the clinician strives to obtain the most significant information possible, while producing the least exposure to the patient. This means that total exposure times should be minimized and that, where adjustable, power should be minimized in exchange for an increase in gain.

CLINICAL STANDARDS FOR THE APPLICATION OF USI IN PHYSIOTHERAPY

Clinical practice standards reflect the minimum level of professional service provided by a professional with regard to a particular application or technique. The suggested standards of practice regarding the use of USI by physiotherapists are:

- All USI equipment must be provincially, state or nationally approved and properly (yearly) maintained.

- Informed consent must be received and recorded by the therapist in the physiotherapy file before an USI assessment or treatment is begun. Patients must be informed that consent can be withdrawn at any time.

- Physiotherapists who employ USI in their clinical practice must have the qualifications to do so. This criterion should be outlined by the licensing body of the physiotherapist's jurisdiction.

- A comprehensive physiotherapy regime for assessment and treatment augmented by USI should include a preliminary physical assessment to determine if USI evaluation is appropriate. If deemed so, then the entire regime should include a history, scanning and biomechanical examination, a USI assessment, education and lifestyle modification, treatment augmented by biofeedback provided by USI and a home exercise programme.

In general, physiotherapists or other rehabilitation professionals who wish to employ USI in their practice require specialized knowledge and skills that are not traditionally acquired in their post-secondary programmes. As such, there is a need for additional training and accreditation. The format, curriculum and instruction of the accreditation process will be dependent upon the specific nature of the licensing jurisdiction of the rehabilitation professional and their practice. For further information on the generic requirements of such an accreditation process the reader is referred to Appendix B.

2 Image generation

In the last decade there has been considerable growth in the knowledge base that serves as the foundation for neuromusculoskeletal rehabilitation. In particular, extensive focus has been placed upon identifying the neuromuscular mechanisms consistent with health, and the specific alterations that underlie dysfunction. From this work it has become evident that a primary impairment underlying dysfunctions such as low-back and pelvic-girdle pain, as well as incontinence, is one of altered neuromuscular control, as opposed to decreased strength or functional capacity (Deindl et al 1994, Jull & Richardson 2000, Barbic et al 2003, Hodges & Moseley 2003, Richardson et al 2004, Cholewicki et al 2005, Stuge et al 2006a). Specifically, there appears to be a trend of evidence consistent with augmented activity of the superficial and diminished activity of the deep muscles of the region (Shirado et al 1995, Zedka et al 1999, Jull & Richardson 2000, Ng et al 2002, Hodges & Moseley 2003, van Dieën et al 2003, Richardson et al 2004).

The deep muscles, which have their origin or insertion on the vertebra or bony pelvis, are commonly referred to as the 'local system' (Bergmark 1989). In the lumbopelvic region this group of muscles has been shown to be both anatomically and neurophysiologically suited to a simultaneous role in respiration, continence and postural control due in part to their ability to influence intra-abdominal pressure (IAP), as well as tension the ligamentous stocking which surrounds the vertebral column and pelvis (Goldman et al 1987, Hodges & Gandevia 2000b, Sapsford 2004, Hodges et al 2005). As these muscles lie deep inside the body their contraction cannot be viewed directly from the surface. The value of USI is that it allows for dynamic study (real-time images) of these deep muscles, as well as the influence they have on the fascial system and adjacent organs, as they contract (Hides et al 1995b, Stokes et al

1997, Whittaker 2004a, b). Hence the complementary use of USI can enhance the clinical analysis of the myofascial system in situations where postural control, respiration or continence are compromised, and has been advocated by various authors (Hides et al 1995b, Dietz et al 2001, Richardson et al 2004, Whittaker 2004a, b).

Several muscles have been nominated for inclusion into the deep or local system, based upon specific neurophysiological (non-direction-specific, early, tonic coactivation to an identifiable perturbation) (Hodges 2003) and anatomical characteristics (extensive attachment into the deep fascia of the lumbopelvic region). The most established of the group are the transversus abdominis (TrA) (Hodges & Richardson 1997, Hodges et al 2003b), the segmental fibres of lumbar multifidus (dMF) (Moseley et al 2002), the diaphragm (Hodges et al 1997, Hodges & Gandevia 2000a, b, Hodges et al 2003b) and the pelvic floor muscles (PFM) (Constantinou & Govan 1982, Bø & Stein 1994, Sapsford et al 2001, Sapsford & Hodges 2001, Barbic et al 2003) (**Fig. 2.1**). Other muscles such as the posterior fibres of psoas major, medial fibres of quadratus lumborum, deep sacral fibres of gluteus maximus and the horizontal fibres of internal oblique have also been considered (Bergmark 1989, O'Sullivan 2000, McGill 2002, Gibbons 2001, 2004). USI has been established as an effective assessment tool for the four established muscles (DeTroyer et al 1990, McKenzie & Gandevia 1994, Hides et al 1995a, Dietz et al 2002), while applications are emerging that consider psoas, quadratus lumborum and deep sacral fibres of gluteus maximus.

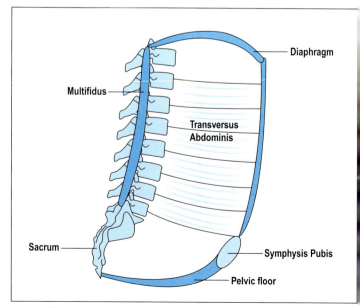

Figure 2.1 The muscles of the lumbopelvic local system.

The use of USI for the assessment of the myofascial system involves three steps; image generation, recognition and interpretation. This chapter will outline the specifics of *image generation* and *recognition* for applications, including:

- The muscles of the lateral abdominal wall and linea semilunaris (transverse view)
- The medial rectus abdominis (RA), midline abdominal fascia and linea alba (transverse view)
- The lumbar multifidus (sagittal and transverse views)
- The bladder and the pelvic floor (sagittal and transverse abdominal views).

LATERAL ABDOMINAL WALL MUSCULATURE

Instrumentation:

Imaging of the lateral abdominal wall is commonly achieved with a 5 MHz curved (convex), or linear array probe, with the ultrasound unit set in B mode (DeTroyer et al 1990, Ferreira et al 2004).

Patient position:

In an attempt to standardize the technique and to facilitate access to the abdomen, a supine, crook-lying position in which the hips are relaxed, and the legs are supported by a bolster is suggested. The abdomen should be exposed from the xyphoid to below the umbilicus (preferably to the symphysis pubis). It is important to consider that this position is used for standardization purposes and is not always the optimal position for assessment or training purposes.

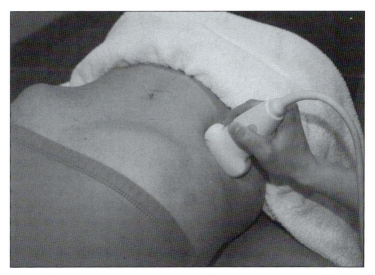

Figure 2.2 Ultrasound probe placement for USI of the lateral abdominal wall muscles.

Probe placement:

The ultrasound probe is placed in a transverse orientation on the anterolateral aspect of the abdominal wall halfway between the iliac crest and inferior border of the rib cage (**Fig. 2.2**). The angle of the probe is manipulated until there is a clear transverse image of all three lateral abdominal muscles (TrA, internal and external oblique) (**Fig. 2.3a, b**). All ultrasound probes have a light or marker on one side that corresponds to a marker on the left side of the ultrasound screen to help orientate the viewer. In this application, the marker is used to orientate patient left (e.g. keep the marker facing the left side of the patient).

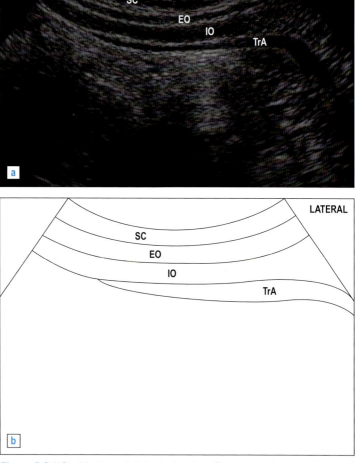

Figure 2.3 USI of the lateral abdominal wall. **a.** Transverse ultrasound image of the right anterolateral abdominal wall. **b.** Labelled outline. SC = subcutaneous tissue, EO = external oblique, IO = internal oblique, TrA = transversus abdominis.

Once the image has been generated the near gain and depth controls can be adjusted to enhance the definition of the muscle and fascial layers, and to ensure that these superficial structures fill approximately 40-50% of the display. The medial to lateral placement of the probe can be manipulated so that both the anterior medial border (linea semilunaris) and the lateral reach of TrA are within the field of view. Although inward probe pressure may maximize the field of view one must consider that this will distort the depth of the lateral abdominal wall muscles. Alternatively, adequate use of ultrasound gel increases the area of contact and minimizes the need for this pressure.

THE MIDLINE ABDOMINAL FASCIA

Instrumentation:

Imaging of the midline abdominal fascia and linea alba is commonly achieved with a 5 MHz curved (convex) or 7.5 linear array probe with the ultrasound unit set in B mode (van Uchelen et al 2001, Whittaker 2004b).

Patient position:

In an attempt to standardize the technique and to facilitate access to the abdomen, a supine, crook-lying position in which the hips are relaxed, and legs supported by a bolster is suggested. The abdomen should be exposed from the xyphoid to below the umbilicus (preferably to the symphysis pubis).

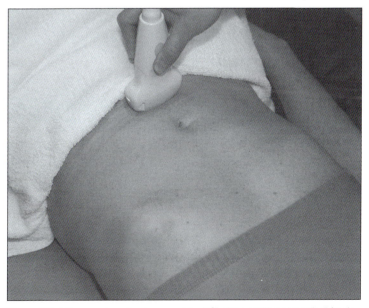

Figure 2.4 Ultrasound probe placement for USI of the midline abdominal fascia.

Probe placement:

The ultrasound probe is placed transversely across the midline of the abdomen at the level of interest (**Fig. 2.4**). The angle of the probe is manipulated (as near vertical as possible) until there is a clear transverse image of the two heads of RA as they meet in the midline (linea alba), as well as the external oblique (EO) and TrA fascia (**Fig. 2.5a, b**). In this application, the marker on the ultrasound probe should be orientated to patient left.

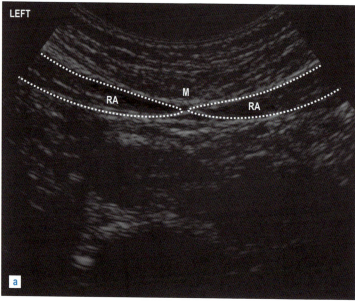

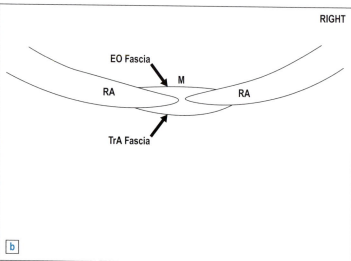

Figure 2.5 USI of the midline abdominal fascia. **a.** Transverse ultrasound image of midline abdominal fascia (above the umbilicus). **b.** Labelled outline. M = midline (linea alba), RA = rectus abdominis, EO = external oblique, TrA = transversus abdominis.

Once the image has been generated, the depth control can be adjusted to ensure that the muscle layers fill approximately 40–50% of the screen, while the medial to lateral placement of the probe can be manipulated so that the linea alba is positioned in the middle of the screen. Delineation of the RA can be challenging. Both lowering the general gain of the ultrasound unit (allowing for the borders of the muscles to become more evident) and asking the patient to lift their head and shoulders off of the bed (producing a contraction and corresponding architectural change within the muscle) can be helpful. Although inward probe pressure may maximize the field of view, one must consider that this will distort the depth of RA. Alternatively, adequate use of ultrasound gel increases the area of contact and minimizes the need for this pressure.

LUMBAR MULTIFIDUS – SAGITTAL APPLICATION

Instrumentation:

Sagittal imaging of the lumbar multifidus is commonly achieved with either a 7 MHz linear array (Hides et al 1995a) or a 5 MHz curved (convex) array probe (Coldron et al 2003, Whittaker 2004b, Stokes et al 2005) with the ultrasound unit set in B mode.

Patient position:

In an attempt to standardize the technique and to optimize feedback for the patient from the ultrasound screen, the suggested position is side-lying with the hips and knees comfortably flexed and the lumbar spine positioned in neutral (Coldron et al 2003). If there is large discrepancy between the hip and waist circumference, a folded towel or pillow should be placed at the waist angle in an attempt to prevent side flexion of the region. The trunk should be exposed so that the abdomen, lower rib cage and vertebral column from the mid-thoracic spine to the sacrum are visible. It is important to consider that this position is used for standardization purposes and is not always the optimal position for assessment or training purposes.

Probe placement:

The ultrasound probe is placed in a sagittal orientation immediately lateral to the spinous process (over the articular pillar) of the level of interest. To visualize multifidus the probe is angled slightly medial, aiming towards the sulcus between the transverse and spinous processes (**Fig. 2.6**). The marker on the probe (indicating the left side of the screen) is orientated towards the patient's head, and the angle of the probe is manipulated until a clear sagittal view of the lumbar multifidus, sacrum and articular processes of L5–S1, L4-5 and L3-4 is achieved (**Fig. 2.7a, b**).

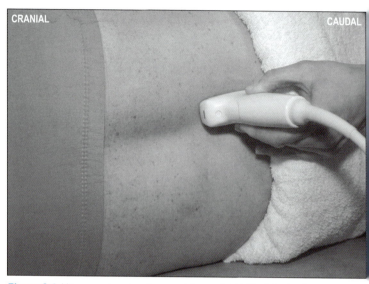

CRANIAL

CAUDAL

Figure 2.6 Ultrasound probe placement for sagittal USI of the lumbar multifidus.

Once the image has been generated, the gain and depth controls can be adjusted to enhance the definition of the muscle/bone interface, and to ensure that multifidus and the spinal column make up the majority of the image displayed on the screen. The delineation between the deep and superficial fibres of the lumbar multifidus is not as obvious as with the layers of the abdominal muscles. The deep fibres of multifidus are located near the articular pillar and the superficial fibres are near the top of the screen. A functional delineation becomes more obvious as a contraction is observed.

LUMBAR MULTIFIDUS – TRANSVERSE APPLICATION

Instrumentation:

Transverse imaging of lumbar multifidus is commonly achieved with a 5 MHz curved (convex) array probe with the ultrasound unit set in B mode (Stokes et al 2005) (**Fig. 2.8**).

Patient position:

The patient can be positioned in either a prone or side-lying position (Hides et al 1995a, Coldron et al 2003, Stokes et al 2005) for this imaging application. However, it is important that the posture of the region is standardized, and that the lumbar spine is positioned in neutral. If prone is chosen, and an obvious lordosis of the thoracolumbar or lumbosacral junction exists, a thin pillow should be placed under the abdomen. The trunk should be exposed so that the entire region is visible. It is important to consider that this position is used for standardization purposes and is not always the optimal position for assessment or training purposes.

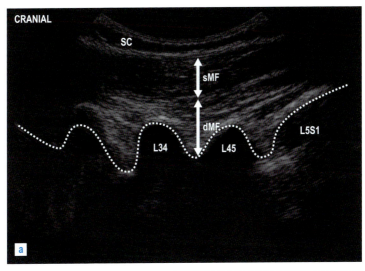

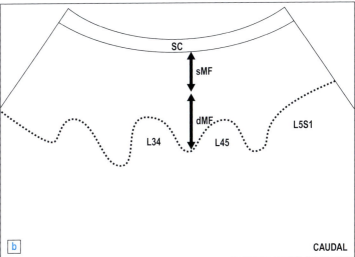

Figure 2.7 USI of lumbar multifidus (sagittal). **a.** Sagittal ultrasound image of lumbar multifidus. **b.** Labelled outline. L34, L45, L5S1 = articular processes, sMF = superficial multifidus, dMF = deep multifidus, SC = subcutaneous tissue.

Probe placement:

Initially the ultrasound probe is placed longitudinally, as in the sagittal application, to determine the level of interest. Once the level of interest is identified, the probe is rotated 90° so that it sits transversely on midline at that vertebral level. In this application, orientate the marker on the probe to patient right (i.e. keep the marker facing the right side of the patient). Once the spinous process of the vertebral level of interest has been identified, the probe can be translated laterally (to highlight the side of interest) and its angle manipulated (**Fig. 2.8**) (slightly anterolateral) until

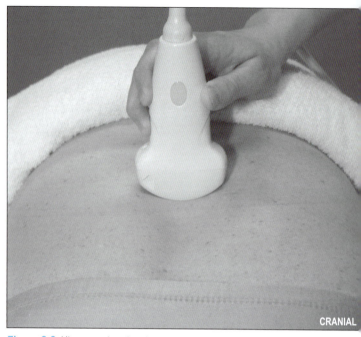

CRANIAL

Figure 2.8 Ultrasound probe placement for transverse USI of the lumbar multifidus.

a clear transverse view of the medial compartment of the lumbar fascia (multifidus), the lamina and spinous process is achieved (**Fig. 2.9a, b**).

It is difficult to delineate the borders (particularly the lateral) of the medial compartment of the lumbar fascia (which contains the multifidus muscle). Both lowering the total gain of the ultrasound unit (so that the borders become more evident) and asking the patient to perform a gentle lift of the ipsilateral leg (Stokes et al 2005) (producing a contraction and corresponding architectural change which will clarify the lateral border of multifidus from longissimus) can be helpful. Once the borders are identified, the depth control can be adjusted so that the multifidus and spinal column make up the majority of the image displayed on the screen. The transverse view allows for differentiation between the medial and intermediate compartments of the lumbar fascia and it is generally used to comment upon symmetry of size and shape, and linear and cross-sectional area measurements, as well as for needle guidance in the laboratory.

BLADDER/PELVIC FLOOR – SAGITTAL APPLICATION

Instrumentation:

Sagittal imaging of the bladder is commonly achieved with a 5 MHz curved (convex) array probe with the ultrasound unit set in B

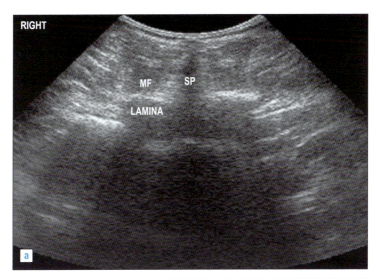

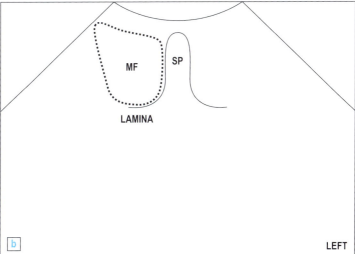

Figure 2.9 USI of lumbar multifidus (transverse). **a.** Transverse ultrasound image of lumbar multifidus. **b.** Labelled outline. SP = spinous process. MF = multifidus.

mode (O'Sullivan et al 2002, Bø et al 2003, Thompson & O'Sullivan 2003, Whittaker 2004a, b).

Patient position:

To standardize the technique and to facilitate access to the lower abdomen, the patient is positioned supine with their legs straight and the hips relaxed. The patient's abdomen should be exposed from the xyphoid to the symphysis pubis. For optimal imaging the bladder needs to be moderately full. This can be achieved by asking the patient to void approximately one hour prior to the assessment, to then drink 500 ml of water, and refrain from voiding until after the assessment is completed. It is important to note that unlike other abdominal ultrasound scans (such as those associated with more traditional imaging goals) where the bladder needs to be near full capacity to serve as an acoustic window, overfilling in this situation will actually confound the assessment process by increasing the resting tone of the PFM.

Probe placement:

The ultrasound probe is placed in a sagittal orientation along the midline of the abdomen with the marker on the probe (indicating the left side of the screen) towards the patient's head. The probe is then translated inferiorly until it encounters the superior aspect of the symphysis pubis. At this point the angle of the probe is manipulated until it is pointing posterior and inferior to the symphysis pubis (towards the gluteal border of the bladder) allowing for a clear image of the bladder and the proximal aspect of its neck (**Fig. 2.11a, b**). If there is interest in one side of the pelvic floor the probe should be further orientated in a slight superolateral to inferomedial direction, just lateral to midline (**Fig. 2.10**).

Once the image has been generated, the gain and depth controls can be adjusted to enhance the definition of the borders of the bladder, and to ensure that the bladder and the structures sitting inferior fill approximately 70% of the screen. Although inward probe pressure may maximize the field of view, one must consider that this will distort the shape of the RA and bladder. Alternatively,

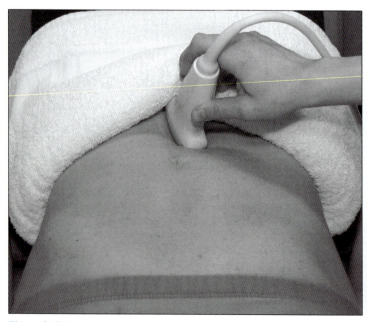

Figure 2.10 Ultrasound probe placement for sagittal USI of the bladder.

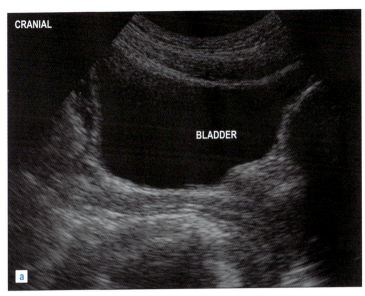

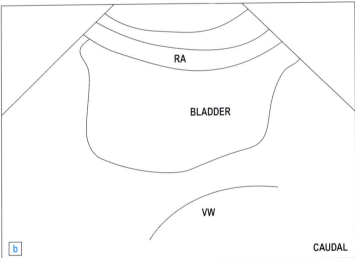

Figure 2.11 USI of the bladder and pelvic floor (sagittal). **a.** Sagittal ultrasound image of the bladder. **b.** Labelled outline. RA = rectus abdominis, BN = neck of the bladder, VW = vaginal wall.

adequate use of ultrasound gel increases the area of contact and minimizes the need for this pressure.

BLADDER/PELVIC FLOOR – TRANSVERSE APPLICATION

Instrumentation:

Transverse imaging of the bladder is commonly achieved with a 5 MHz curved (convex) array probe with the ultrasound unit set in B mode (Whittaker 2004a, b, Sherburn et al 2005).

Patient position:

In an attempt to standardize the technique and to facilitate access to the lower abdomen, the patient is placed in a supine position with their hips relaxed and legs supported by a bolster. The patient's abdomen should be exposed from the xyphoid to the symphysis pubis. As with the sagittal application the bladder needs to be moderately full (300–500 ml).

Probe placement:

The ultrasound probe is placed in a transverse orientation, across the midline of the abdomen, immediately superior to the pubic symphysis. The angle of the probe is manipulated until it is approximately 60° from the vertical and aimed towards the gluteal or posteroinferior region of the bladder (**Fig. 2.12**). The marker on the probe (indicating the left side of the display screen) should be orientated towards the left side of the patient. The angle of the probe should be adjusted until there is a clear image of the bladder and the midline pelvic floor structures (urethra, perineal body, rectum etc.) as seen in **Fig. 2.13a, b** (Whittaker 2004a).

Once the image has been generated the gain and depth controls can be adjusted to enhance the definition of the borders of the bladder, and to ensure that the bladder and the structures sitting inferior fill approximately 70% of the screen. Although inward

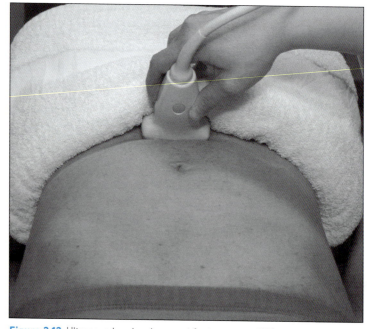

Figure 2.12 Ultrasound probe placement for transverse USI of the bladder.

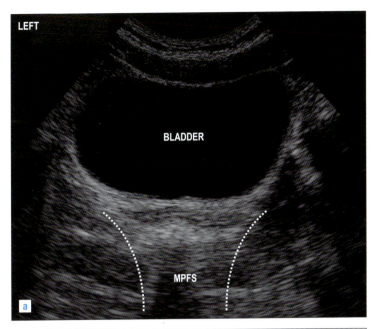

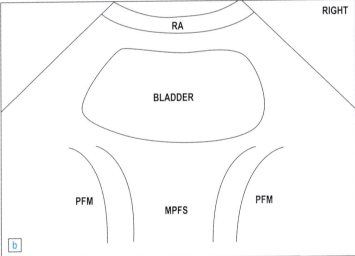

Figure 2.13 USI of the bladder and pelvic floor (transverse). **a.** Transverse ultrasound image of the urinary bladder and pelvic floor. **b.** Labelled outline. RA = rectus abdominis, PFM = pelvic floor muscles, MPFS = midline pelvic floor structures.

probe pressure may maximize the field of view, one must consider that this will distort the shape of the RA and bladder. Alternatively, adequate use of ultrasound gel increases the area of contact and minimizes the need for this pressure.

GENERAL IMAGING CONSIDERATIONS

The practicalities involved in generating the images outlined in this chapter are relatively uncomplicated. However, as with all skill acquisition, and in particular for individuals new to ultrasound technology, there is a learning curve. The following are worthwhile considerations which will facilitate the process.

Ultrasound unit orientation:

● If the patient is in a supine position the ultrasound unit should be placed to one side and orientated such that it faces the patient. The therapist should sit to this side of the patient, facing the ultrasound unit. The hand closest to the patient should be used to control the ultrasound probe, leaving the other free to manipulate the unit and to bring attention to the structures and happenings on the display (**Fig. 2.14a**).

● If the patient is in a side-lying position the ultrasound unit should be placed in front of them to facilitate their view of the display. The therapist can sit behind the patient and still be capable of both manipulating the ultrasound probe, and bringing attention to the happenings on the display (**Fig. 2.14b**). If the display screen is too far away to reach then a small laser pointer can be used to bring attention to the structures and various happenings.

● If possible the patient should be brought to the height of the therapist's imaging arm.

Ultrasound probe practicalities:

● To optimize image quality, care must be taken to ensure maximal penetration of the ultrasound wave. Consequently, it is critical to eliminate all air between the ultrasound probe and the patient's skin. This is accomplished by adequate application of ultrasound gel to the surface of the probe as opposed to the region of the body that is to be imaged. If one area has been imaged (e.g. the lower abdominal wall) and the probe is being moved to another (e.g. the lateral abdominal wall) then the gel will also have to be moved or reapplied to the probe if the quality of the image is to be retained.

● During the initial stages of image generation the ultrasound probe should be held with an overhand grip in the hand closest to the patient. The value of the overhand grip is that it prevents the therapist's hand from getting caught between the probe and the patient's body when the angle of the probe is being manipulated. This is particularly useful with the bladder and pelvic floor imaging applications.

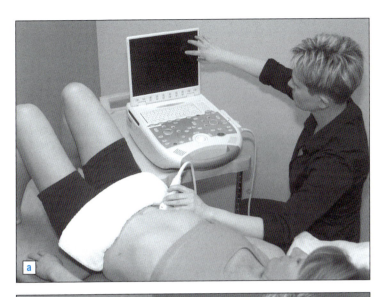

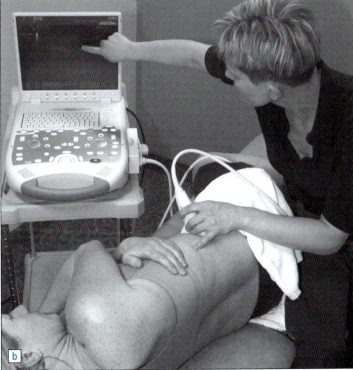

Figure 2.14 Ultrasound unit orientation. **a.** Patient, therapist and ultrasound unit orientation for supine imaging applications. **b.** Patient, therapist and ultrasound unit orientation for side-lying imaging applications.

- The therapist should always attend to the position of the probe on the patient's body before looking at the ultrasound display. This will facilitate the orientation process and cut down on the amount of time spent manipulating the probe position. Once the probe is appropriately positioned on the patient the therapist can then look at the display and make the minor adjustments that are required to 'focus in' on the area of interest.

- The angle of the ultrasound probe can be adjusted to improve the definition of tissue boundaries and optimize the displayed image (e.g. increase the amount of ultrasound that is encountering the boundary at 90°) by tilting it in either a cranial/caudal or medial/lateral direction. When making these minor adjustments in probe orientation it is important to move the probe slowly, only a degree at a time, as quick surface movements result in large amplitude jumps deeper, and a loss of the structure of interest.

- Once the ideal image has been achieved, the therapist can reposition their imaging hand on the probe (**Fig. 2.14a, b**) in such a way that they rest both the ulnar aspect of their hand and a portion of the ulnar aspect of their forearm on the patient in an attempt to steady the probe during the assessment process. The stability of the probe can be further facilitated by resting the elbow of the imaging arm on the stationary surface of the bed or plinth. Failure to steady the probe may result in movement of the probe with respect to the body surface and result in motion and architectural changes in the structures within the ultrasound image that may be misinterpreted.

In an attempt to master the skills associated with image generation and recognition, therapists are encouraged to practice generating images on individuals with a variety of body types and, as their skills improve, in a variety of postures (seated, standing, four-point kneel etc.). To expedite skill acquisition the initial focus should centre entirely upon image generation and recognition without concentration being diverted to the interpretation process.

3 Image interpretation: qualitative

It is well accepted that USI is a tool capable of establishing both muscle size and activity (DeTroyer et al 1990, Hides et al 1992, Coldron et al 2003, Bø et al 2003, Hodges et al 2003a, Thompson & O'Sullivan 2003, Ferreira et al 2004, McMeeken et al 2004, Stokes et al 2005, Thompson et al 2005a, Hides et al 2006). However, there are limitations to the information that the technology can provide and their careful consideration is essential as it ensures appropriate interpretation and accurate reporting (Hodges et al 2003a, Ferreria et al 2004, Hodges 2005a, Thompson et al 2005).

Most USI applications reported in the literature are quantitative in nature and provide a measure of width, depth, length, cross-sectional area, or volume from a static image. The accurate analysis of static ultrasound images is limited primarily by the ability to anatomically orientate oneself, and methodological practicalities such as consistent definition of measurement site, muscle boundaries, as well as probe placement, orientation, and inward pressure. However, extrapolating that an increase in an architectural measure (e.g. depth) of a muscle is indicative of actual activity may be presumptuous, as the relationship between the two is complex and inconsistent (Hodges et al 2003a, Hodges 2005a). The potential for a discrepancy exists due to the nature and limitations of two-dimensional imaging (e.g. a muscle contraction produces architectural changes in three dimensions as opposed to the two dimensions visible on an ultrasound display), as well as the potential for a change in architecture in the presence of a competing force on the muscle (e.g. protrusion of the abdominal contents during respiration may impact the depth of the abdominal wall muscles). Furthermore, factors such as initial muscle length, width, as well as the pennation pattern of the muscle can potentially impact architectural change and must also be taken into consideration (Hodges 2005a). Nevertheless, if these issues are considered, and appropriate care is taken (see Chapter 4), accurate analysis and measurement is possible (Hodges et al 2003a, Bunce et al 2004, Stokes et al 2005, Teyher et al 2005, Whittaker 2005, Hides et al 2006).

Ultimately, the use of USI to describe a muscle contraction is a complex issue. Although changes in static architectural parameters tell a portion of the story, considered alone they primarily reflect muscle capacity, and infer that 'more is better'. If the clinical and scientific interest in the musculature system is related to altered neuromuscular control, it is imperative that more-encompassing methods of describing what is being seen on the ultrasound display are developed. Considering only the increase in an architectural parameter of a muscle during a task is analogous to considering the maximal amount of EMG activity without taking into account timing, or influence on other structures. Consequently, it is the strong belief of this author that in addition to the measurement of quantitative parameters (Chapter 4) there is a role for qualitative analysis of the dynamic features that occur when a muscle contracts. For instance, commenting on the simultaneous vs. independent or, phasic vs. sustained increase in depth of a muscle, or group of muscles, with a task, as well as the ability of the muscles to relax once the task ceases, proves invaluable in the clinical interpretation of a neuromuscular strategy. Although components of qualitative analysis have been proposed by several authors (Richardson et al 2004, Whittaker 2004a, b) the incorporation of such parameters into the scientific setting is complicated, hence has been limited.

This chapter will demonstrate how vigilant use of the applications outlined in Chapter 2 combined with a knowledge base regarding postural control of the trunk, respiration and continence will allow one to ascertain (through qualitative analysis) if an individual can produce and maintain a coordinated, isometric, low-intensity co-contraction of the deep muscles in the lumbopelvic region, and sustain it during loading activities. Additionally, these applications will be used to speculate on muscle tissue quality and resting tone, as well as the ability of the endopelvic and midline abdominal fascia to transmit tension. Image interpretation is unique for each and will be discussed separately.

An evaluation process should be founded upon sound clinical reasoning, such that the order and number of procedures chosen for a specific patient vary depending on the explicit needs and concerns of that individual. The ability to demonstrate clinical reasoning is dependent upon a multitude of factors, including clinician experience and knowledge base. Throughout this chapter an attempt will be made to provide a basis for determining when these applications should be employed, and how the information that is attained can be used to direct further assessment and ultimately, treatment. However, until the therapist has attained the experience and knowledge to streamline the assessment process they may benefit from an inclusive blueprint for the USI assessment process (refer to Appendix A).

INTERNAL OBLIQUE (IO) AND TRANSVERSUS ABDOMINIS (TrA)

There is some debate concerning the correlation between the amount of architectural change (depth, width and length) seen in the lateral abdominal wall muscles (external oblique, internal oblique and transversus abdominis) during a contraction, and the actual muscle activity present. Hodges et al (2003a) noted, during an isometric contraction of TrA and IO, that the increase in depth and decrease in length seen on USI exhibited a non-linear relationship with actual muscle activity, measured by indwelling electromyography ($n = 3$). Furthermore, they determined that contractions between 12 and 23% of maximal voluntary contraction (MVC) produced the most significant architectural changes. In contrast, McMeeken et al (2004) demonstrated a linear relationship between increases in depth of TrA and indwelling EMG activity in a slightly larger group of subjects ($n = 9$). Although the studies differ in their conclusions regarding the ability of USI to discriminate between moderate and strong contractions (>40% MVC), they concur that architectural changes detected with USI are sensitive to the submaximal contractions (less than 20-30% MVC) which are being discussed in this text. Furthermore, these and a previous study (Ninane et al 1992) identified inconsistent changes in the depth of external oblique (EO) with this imaging approach and concluded that measurements of this muscle from this plane of view cannot be used to accurately detect activity.

Clinically, there are four goals associated with imaging the muscles of the lateral abdominal wall. The first is related to resting state, the next two consider automatic activation, and the fourth is dependent upon voluntary effort:

1. Speculate on the resting state and shape of TrA and IO.

2. Determine the impact of resting respiration on the architecture of TrA and IO.

3. Determine if TrA and IO demonstrate sustained tonic activity during a task that loads the spine and pelvis, such as an active straight leg raise (ASLR), and then fully relax after the challenge.

4. Determine if TrA can be preferentially activated. Specifically contracted in relative isolation from the superficial abdominal musculature (IO, EO and RA), and maintained as an isometric low-intensity contraction that results in fascial tensioning and co-contraction of the other local system (PFM, diaphragm and the dMF) muscles.

Resting state

A variety of studies have reported on the motor control change seen with regard to the superficial muscles of the trunk in individuals with low-back pain (LBP) (Shirado et al 1995, Zedka et al 1999, Ng et al 2002). The results are variable but there appears to be consistent evidence suggestive of augmented activity (Hodges & Moseley 2003, van Dieën et al 2003). Although there is no evidence to date which would indicate that an increase in resting muscle tone is detectable with USI, clinical experience has revealed that several qualitative characteristics seen within a resting ultrasound image correlate with clinical indicators of hypertonicity. These clinical indicators include the presence of trigger points and taut bands within a muscle, decreased muscle length, corresponding loss in range of motion and intolerance to further compression or weight-bearing through the region. Consequently, once an image of the lateral abdominal wall (**Fig. 2.3a, b**) has been generated the resting architecture and relationship of the muscle layers and their fascia should be considered.

Although there is individual variability, a normal resting image of the lateral abdominal wall is characterized by muscle layers that are tapered in depth towards their anterior medial reach (linea semilunaris), essentially even in their middle region, and display a slight corset laterally (**Fig. 3.1a**). Urquhart et al (2005) have shown that in the region between the bottom of the rib cage and the top of the iliac crest, both the IO and external oblique (EO) are generally thicker than TrA, with IO being significantly thicker than EO.

In contrast, a muscle layer(s) that has increased resting tone (hypertonic) is enlarged, more equal in depth, and often broaden into its anterior medial reach (linea semilunaris). Furthermore, the hypertonic layer(s) is commonly held in a fixed corset shape (arc at its lateral reach and has a characteristic appearance of protruding into its fascia and adjacent muscle layers, analogous to a sausage casing filled beyond its capacity (**Fig. 3.1b**). The presumption of resting hypertonicity is further legitimized if either a voluntarily or involuntarily relaxation of the muscle in question is seen during the examination process and the corresponding architectural change are noted or, if the image can be compared to what is believed to be a 'normal' contralateral abdominal wall.

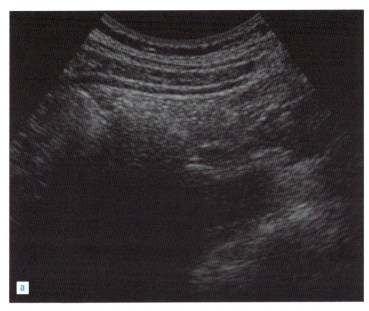

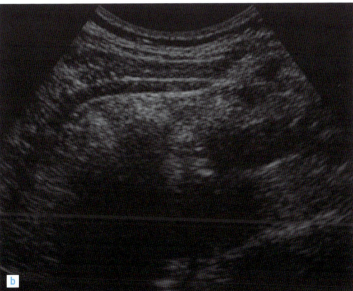

Figure 3.1 USI of the lateral abdominal wall – resting state. **a.** Normal resting ultrasound image of the left anterolateral abdominal wall. **b.** Hypertonic resting image of the left anterolateral abdominal wall demonstrating hypertonicity of both TrA and IO. Note the thickness and protruding nature, as well as the lateral corset of both muscles.

Resting respiration

Once the resting state of the lateral abdominal wall muscles has been considered, the next step in the assessment process is to observe for any fluctuations in their architecture during resting supine respiration. Several investigators have indicated that the activity of the middle fibres of TrA should be minimal during quiet breathing, and that no obvious activity should be detected in IO (Strohl et al 1981, Goldman et al 1987, DeTroyer et al 1990, Ninane et al 1992). However, in situations in which there is either an increase in respiratory drive (either chemical or behavioural) or elastic loading through the thorax (due to a thoracic joint fixation, disease process or hypertonicity of the superficial muscles), TrA (followed by IO) is the first abdominal muscle recruited to assist expiration (**Fig. 3.2a, b**) (DeTroyer et al 1990, Ninane et al 1992, Abe et al 1996, Misuri et al 1997, Hodges et al 2001). Therefore, a modulated contraction (increase in depth, decrease in length) of TrA (or IO) corresponding to expiration, during quiet breathing, is a potential indicator of hyperactivity of the muscle and/or concurrent breathing dysfunction (**Fig. 3.2a, b**) (Whittaker 2005).

As the architecture of the lateral abdominal wall during quiet supine respiration is monitored it is critical to remember that muscle tissue is encapsulated within a fascial stocking of fixed volume, similar to water in a balloon. Hence, pressure into the muscle layers by the expanding abdomen during inspiration will result in thinning of the muscle layer and portray a change in depth which may be falsely mistaken for activity as the muscle returns to its resting depth during expiration. Hence, great diligence must be taken to monitor both length and depth changes as well as the frequency, depth and predominant pattern of respiration (e.g. apical, lateral costal or abdominal) of the patient. Whittaker (2005) has shown that an average increase in TrA depth of <1.3% (±5.8%) and IO of <2% (±7.2%) with respiration should be considered normal in a lumbopelvic dysfunction population, while an average increase in the depth of TrA greater than 20% correlates highly with the coexistence of hypocapnia (Gardner 1996).

It is important to realize that the identification of breathing dysfunction is a crucial preliminary step in the clinical reasoning process. Specifically, as respiration is a physiological priority, any attempts to restore motor control to the region without attention to the source of the increased respiratory drive and resultant expiratory modulation will likely fail. Consequently, if respiratory modulation is present then the initial focus of clinical management must be aimed at detecting the dysfunction and restoring the mechanics and chemistry of respiration (Chaitow et al 2002, Whittaker 2005).

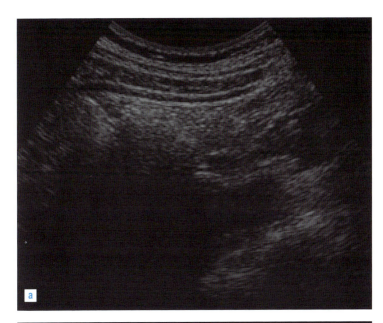

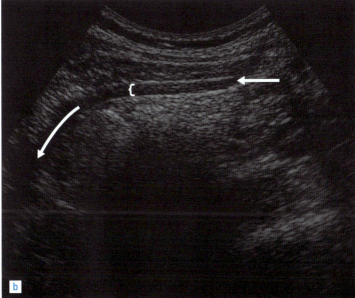

Figure 3.2 USI of the lateral abdominal wall – resting respiratory modulation. **a.** Resting ultrasound image of the left anterolateral abdominal wall at the height of inspiration. **b.** Resting image of the left anterolateral abdominal wall at the end of expiration. Note the increase in depth and decrease in length of the TrA, as well as the lateral corset of both the TrA and IO.

Tonic activity with spinal loading

After the abdominal musculature has been monitored at rest and during quiet respiration, the patient is asked to perform a task that loads the spine such as a resisted arm lift, ASLR (from a supine position lift the extended leg 5 cm off the supporting surface) (Mens et al 2001, Lee 2004) or a modified active leg raise (from a supine crook lie position lift one leg maintaining a flexed knee) (Ferreira et al 2004) (**Fig. 3.3a, b**). Several studies (Hodges et al 1996,

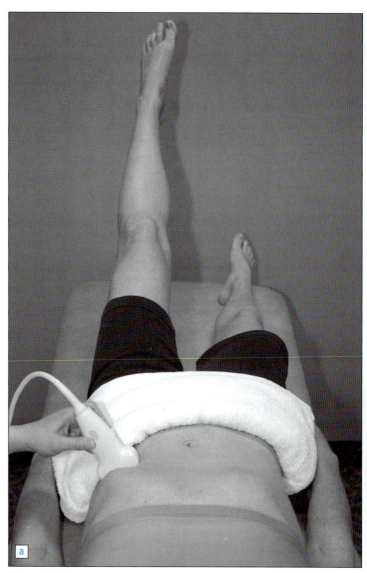

Figure 3.3 Ultrasound probe placement to monitor the lateral abdominal wall muscles during **a.** ASLR.

Hodges & Richardson 1997, Saunders et al 2004) have reported that in a normal population, TrA should contract prior to the superficial lateral abdominal wall muscles and remain tonically active throughout such a task. In contrast delayed and absent activity of TrA has been reported in individuals with LBP (Hodges 2001, Cowan et al 2004, Ferreira et al 2004). Although the pre-activation of TrA is a matter of milliseconds, consequently imperceptible to the naked eye, the tonic activity of TrA during such a task is visible with USI.

When limb motion is initiated, a bilateral contraction of both TrA and IO should be observed. This will be seen as an increase in depth, decrease in length, and lateral corseting (**Fig. 3.4b**) of both TrA and IO in the ultrasound image. The contractions of TrA and

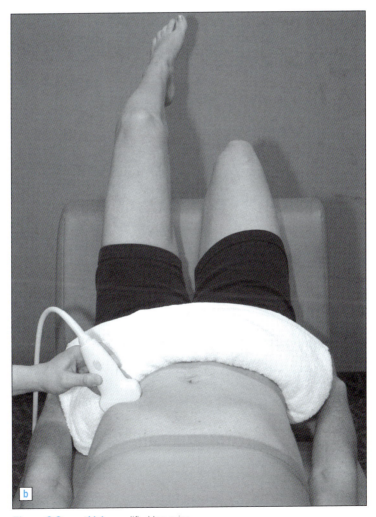

Figure 3.3, cont'd b. modified leg raise.

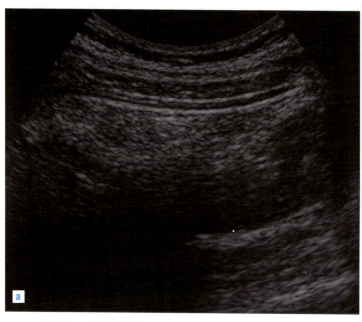

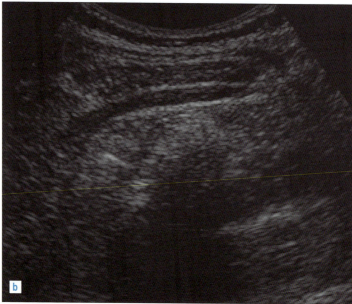

Figure 3.4 USI of the lateral abdominal wall – ASLR (three images taken in sequence). **a.** Resting image of the left lateral abdominal wall. **b.** Optimal co-contraction of the IO and TrA during the initial stages of the ASLR. Note the increase in depth, decrease in length and lateral corset of both muscles.

IO should persist during the entire limb loading task and then fully relax once the leg is lowered. Absence (**Fig. 3.4c**), observable delay or premature loss (e.g. relaxation before the leg is lowered) of these architectural changes, or an excessive response followed by inability to fully relax after the task are considered abnormal. The first three

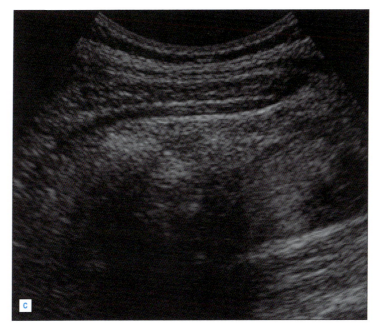

Figure 3.4, cont'd c. Premature relaxation (the leg is still being held off the bed) of both muscles during the later stages of the ASLR.

scenarios indicate a deficiency in either motor control or capacity of the TrA (or its fascia), and the fourth potential hyperactivity.

It is important to realize that RTUS applications that involve significant increases in intra-abdominal pressure (IAP), such as coughing, sneezing or in this case limb motion, require diligent attention to steady the position, orientation and inward pressure of the ultrasound probe. Failure to do so will result in motion of the probe with respect to the body, and false conclusions with regard to muscle behaviour (Pranathi Reddy et al 2001, Whittaker 2004a). In an attempt to control motion and maintain consistent inward pressure of the probe (by matching the outward increase in pressure during the task) the examiner should employ both hands, as well as firmly steady their forearms on the patient's torso and the treatment table.

Preferential activation of transversus abdominis

After commenting on the resting state and monitoring the involuntary activity of TrA and IO during quiet breathing and with a task that loads the spine, the patient is asked to produce a voluntary, relatively isolated, contraction of TrA using one of a variety of verbal commands. It is important to note that at this time there is no published evidence to suggest that an inability to achieve this task is in anyway related to the altered involuntary motor control identified in the literature with regard to individuals with LBP (Stuge et al 2006a). The rationale for assessing the ability to produce an isolated voluntary contraction is based upon clinical experience and extrapolation of the evidence indicating that the deep muscle system is anticipatory and non-direction specific in its activation (Constantinou & Govan 1982, Hodges & Richardson 1997, Hodges & Gandevia 2000a, Hodges et al 2002, Moseley et al 2002). That is, when the central nervous system can anticipate spinal and/or pelvic loading, it increases the activity of these muscles in response. This anticipatory characteristic suggests that the deep muscles have a separate, yet coordinated, control mechanism from that of the superficial musculature. Furthermore, its existence in health, and loss in dysfunction (Richardson et al 2004), necessitates consideration of motor control. Clinically, this involves the evaluation of the ability to access the specific neurological pathways to these muscles and produce a voluntary isolated contraction (in the absence of global muscle activity).

It is critical to realize that preferential activation evaluates many factors beyond the health of the motor control pathways. For instance, the individual's ability and motivation to learn, as well as the ability of the therapist to instruct will have an influence on the success of this task (Hodges 2005a). Hence, there is no magical cue that will elicit the correct contraction. Some common clinical cues include (adapted from Lee 2004):

- 'Slowly and gently draw your lower abdominal wall in towards your spine'.
- 'Slowly and gently contract the muscles that slow the flow of urine'.
- 'Slowly and gently draw your vagina (or testicles) up into your abdomen'.
- 'Slowly and gently think about closing your rear passage (anus)'.

Often there is benefit from kinaesthetic assistance as opposed to, or in addition to, verbal cues. The therapist can use the surface of their hand to encase the lower abdomen, or can protrude their fingers into the lower abdomen to give the patient something to concentrate on. Using a side-lying position, which allows the abdominal contents to fall onto the deep surface of the TrA, can also facilitate kinaesthetic awareness (see Chapter 5).

Definition of an isolated TrA contraction

An ideal response (**Fig. 3.5a, b**) results in a slow and controlled increase in the depth, and decrease in the length, of the TrA with minimal architectural change of the IO. It is important that the TrA corsets or arcs in its lateral aspect, and that the tension in the

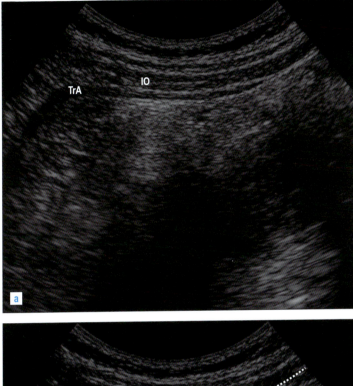

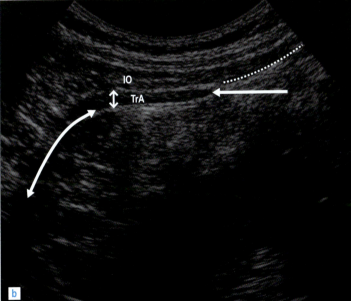

Figure 3.5 USI of the lateral abdominal wall – preferential activation.
a. Resting image of the left lateral abdominal wall **b.** An isolated contraction of TrA; note the isolated increase in depth, and lateral corseting (double curved arrow) as it slides under (horizontal arrow) the IO and increases the tension in the anterior TrA fascia (dotted curved line).

abdominal (linea semilunaris) and lumbar fascia increases as the TrA shortens, sliding under the IO (Richardson et al 2004, Whittaker 2004b, Hides et al 2006). The response, seen on imaging, should be correlated with that noted on palpation (TrA can be palpated through the internal oblique inferior and medial to the ASIS (**Fig. 3.8**).

If the patient is capable of producing an isolated contraction of TrA they are then asked to repeat the contraction and hold it while continuing to breathe. Clinically, there appears to be some correlation between an inability to sustain a tonic TrA contraction while breathing in a coordinated fashion and breathing dysfunction. Hence this is an important consideration as it may indicate that further investigation of the individual's breathing status may be required. If an isolated contraction can be sustained in coordination with breathing, the examiner should concurrently palpate for a co-contraction of the segmental fibres of the lumbosacral multifidus (**Fig. 3.14**). This will establish the endurance capacity of TrA, as well as its ability to coordinate and co-contract with the other muscles of the local system.

Abnormal responses

Abnormal responses include absent or insufficient recruitment of TrA, or an inability to contract the TrA in isolation from the superficial abdominal muscles. As the response is often asymmetrical, both sides of the abdomen should be imaged. It is important to remember that this particular USI application cannot be used to draw conclusions regarding EO activity (Ninane et al 1992, Hodges et al 2003a) due in part to the angle of pennation of this muscle. Consequently, an increase in EO activity will require reorientation of the ultrasound probe, palpation, or use of supplementary surface electromyography (Ng et al 1998).

An absent or insufficient response results in ineffective force closure of the lumbopelvic region and is secondary to a deficiency of the contractile component (absent or hypoactive contraction, altered length tension or atrophy) and/or a loss of integrity of the fascial system (e.g. lengthening or diastasis of the linea alba, or an abdominal hernia) (Lee 2004). Force closure refers to compression produced by the coordinated efforts of muscle, ligament and fascia to augment the structure, orientation and shape of a joint such that optimal load transfer can occur (Vleeming et al 1997, Lee 2004). When the contractile component is insufficient, the fascial system is not sufficiently tensed, and little change will be seen between the resting and contracted images. If the insufficiency is due to fascial lengthening (e.g. post-partum), or disruption (diastasis, hernia) the individual may demonstrate preferential activation; however, an excessive lateral slide of the TrA will be seen in association with disproportionate shortening as the muscle contracts in on itself due to the incompetence of its anterior (linea semilunaris) fascial anchor (**Fig. 3.6a, b**). Another clue pointing to lengthening of the abdominal fascia is an increase in the distance of the anterior reach of TrA with respect to the midline. Clinical experience suggests that this intersection (linea semilunaris) should be at or anterior to the mid-axillary line and that if it is found lateral to this it is likely indicative of lengthened fascia and/or RA.

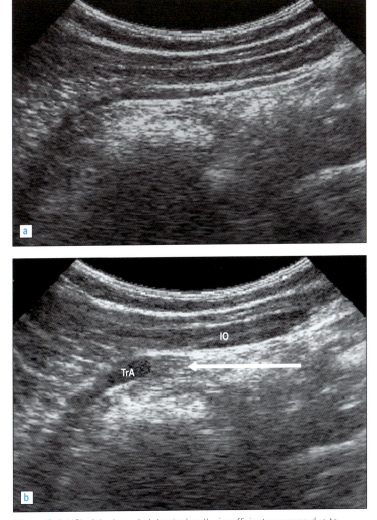

Figure 3.6 USI of the lateral abdominal wall – insufficient response due to altered length tension. **a.** Resting image of the left lateral abdominal wall **b.** An isolated response of TrA in which there appears to be a loss of the anterior fascial anchor at the linea semilunaris. Note the excessive lateral slide (arrow) of TrA under IO as well the disproportionate shortening.

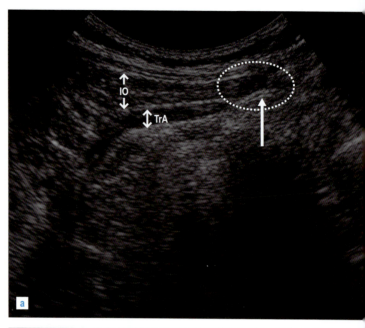

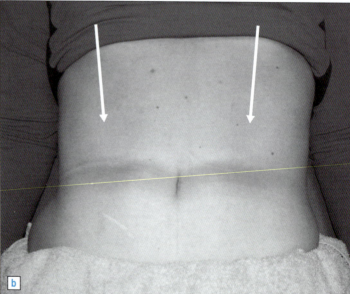

Figure 3.7 USI of the lateral abdominal wall – excessive response.
a. Ultrasound image of the left lateral abdominal wall demonstrating a hyperactive response of IO and TrA. Note the increase in depth of both IO and TrA (double arrows), the lack of disassociation or slide of TrA under IO, and the characteristic protrusion of the anterior reach of the IO into the slack anterior TrA fascia (dotted oval). **b.** Depiction of rib cage depression with thoracopelvic flexion.

An inability to isolate the TrA demonstrated by a simultaneous contraction of the oblique abdominals, or RA, may result in inappropriate (excessive) force closure of the pelvis, lumbar spine and thorax (Lee 2004). The resulting ultrasound image will demonstrate a concurrent, phasic, increase in depth and decrease in length of both the TrA and IO (**Fig. 3.7a**). This simultaneous contraction

TABLE 3.1 OBSERVATIONAL CONSIDERATIONS DURING PREFERENTIAL ACTIVATION OF TRANSVERSUS ABDOMINIS

PHASE	CONSIDERATION	POTENTIAL IMPLICATION
Resting position	Position of the spine (neutral, flexed, extended)	Resting superficial muscle tone
	Location and symmetry of breathing pattern (apical, lateral costal, abdominal)	Degree of abdominal laxity, increased thoracic elasticity (joint dysfunction, muscle hypertonicity, disease process)
	Presence of creases or rib clamping Expiratory activity of the oblique abdominals	Resting superficial muscle tone Underlying breathing dysfunction
	Hernia	Bias towards the use of a high IAP strategy
	Diastasis, stretch marks	Laxity in the myofascial system
	Scars	Adhesions between muscle layers
During contraction	Movement of the spine (thoracolumbar flexion, posterior pelvic tilt, thoracic rotation)	Superficial muscle activity
	Movement of the rib cage (expansion, clamping down, gripping)	Superficial muscle activity
	Visible contraction of the abdominal muscles	Superficial muscle activity
	Upward, downward or outward motion of the umbilicus	Superficial muscle activity, or increased IAP (outward)
	Inward motion of the umbilicus	Potential TrA isolation
	Alteration in breathing pattern (holding, valsalva, bearing down)	Superficial muscle activity, underlying breathing dysfunction
	Speed of contraction (phasic vs. tonic)	Type of muscle activated (phasic = superficial)
During relaxation	Inability to fully relax the abdomen	Hypertonicity
	Speed and coordination of relaxation	State of motor control
	Movement of the spine	Relaxation of superficial muscle activity

will fail to demonstrate the independent sliding (shortening) of the TrA under the IO that is responsible for increasing the tension in the anterior TrA fascia (linea semilunaris). Consequently, a characteristic protrusion of the anterior reach of IO into this fascia will be seen (**Fig. 3.7a**). Additionally, outward pressure of the abdominal wall may be detected through the ultrasound probe and either depression of the rib cage towards the pelvis (thoracolumbar flexion)

TABLE 3.2 PALPATORY CONSIDERATIONS DURING PREFERENTIAL ACTIVATION OF TRANSVERSUS ABDOMINIS

PHASE	CONSIDERATION	POTENTIAL IMPLICATION
Resting position	Quality of resting muscle tone (abdominals, erector spinae etc.)	Possible superficial muscle tone
	Location and symmetry of breathing pattern (apical, lateral costal, abdominal)	Amount of abdominal laxity, increase thoracic elasticity (joint dysfunction, muscle hypertonicity, disease process)
	Freedom of the rib cage to disassociate from the pelvis (resistance to rib cage wiggle)	Degree of resting muscle tone
During contraction	Quality of the tension developed with the contraction (drawing in of the fingers until a lightly tensioned trampoline sensation is felt)	Isolated contraction of the TrA
	Quality of the tension developed with the contraction (fingers being pushed out of the lower abdominal wall)	Oblique abdominal activity and/or increase in IAP
	Movement of the rib cage (feel for rigidity or bracing)	Superficial muscle activity
	Movement of the thoracolumbar junction or rib cage	Superficial muscle activity
	Movement of the pelvis (feel for posterior tilt)	Superficial muscle activity
	Palpable co-contraction of the lumbar multifidus	Local system co-contraction
	Co-contraction of the erector spinae, external rotators of the hip etc.	Superficial muscle activity
During relaxation	Inability to relax the abdomen, status of the resting muscle tone	Hypertonicity
	Speed and coordination of relaxation	State of motor control
	Movement of the spine	Relaxation of superficial muscle activity
	Movement of the pelvis	Relaxation of superficial muscle activity

or posterior tilting of the pelvis (lumbosacral flexion) may be observed (**Fig. 3.7b**).

When USI is used to assess the behaviour of a muscle there is a tendency to focus entirely on the display screen. It is critical that the therapist keep in mind that USI is only an adjunct to the examination process and not to abandon other tools such as observation and palpation. It is critical that the patient is observed and TrA is palpated throughout the ultrasound assessment (**Fig. 3.8**). **Tables 3.1** and **3.2** summarize common observation and palpation considerations and their potential implications.

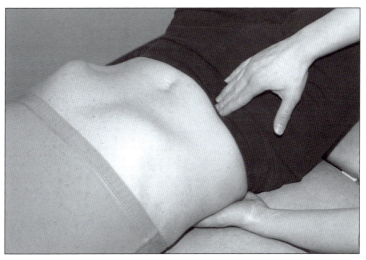

Figure 3.8 Palpation site for TrA (medial and inferior to the ASIS).

MIDLINE ABDOMINAL FASCIA

The integrity of the fascia that extends from, and envelops, the muscles that delineate the boundaries of the abdominal cavity (TrA, the PFM, diaphragm and dMF) is crucial for their function. Anteriorly the transmission of forces produced by TrA will diminish if there is either an increase in width or a loss of structural integrity of the linea alba or abdominal fascia. An increase in width can result from repetitive use of high IAP strategies (either for lumbopelvic postural control or straining with bowel evacuation etc.), obesity or pregnancy, while a loss of fascial integrity is most commonly seen with either diastasis or an abdominal hernia. Clinically, there are two goals associated with USI of the midline abdominal fascia (linea alba). The first is related to resting state, and the second considers the impact of either increasing IAP pressure or muscle activation upon the fascia:

1. Speculate on the resting state, tissue quality and integrity of the RA and midline abdominal fascia (linea alba).

2. Determine if the width of the midline abdominal fascia either decreases (may suggest efficient transmission of tension), increases or is not affected (may suggest inefficient transmission of tension) by activities that result in either activation of the muscles that attach into it (RA, EO, IO and TrA) and/or produce an increase in IAP (head lift, straining, cough, sneeze, active straight or modified leg raise).

Resting state

The integrity of the midline abdominal fascia can be easily established with USI (van Uchelen et al 2001, Whittaker 2004b). Once an appropriate image (**Fig. 2.5a, b**) has been generated, the resting architecture and relationship of the two heads of RA, as well as the intervening fascia, are considered. Attention is paid to the clarity of the muscle contours, as well as the delineation of the layers of the midline fascia. In addition, the echogenicity of the RA with respect to a reference muscle (e.g. if the probe is drawn laterally IO can be brought into the field of view), at a set gain level, can be commented upon. As we will see below, in reference to multifidus, greater echogenicity of a muscle may be associated with an increase in fatty and fibrous content, which can occur with ageing, chronic disuse (Tsubahara et al 1995, Campbell et al 2005) or denervation as a result of an injury (Andary et al 1998). Although there are no references with respect to fatty infiltration of RA in the literature, increases in echogenicity have been seen clinically. However, when interpreting the ultrasound image it is important to note that the midline abdominal region is a common site for adipose tissue and consequently it is possible to see a great deal of scatter (**Fig. 1.5a**) which may change the appearance of the ultrasound image (e.g. increase the echogenicity) and lead to false conclusions regarding tissue quality.

Response to load

After the integrity, clarity and echogenicity of RA and midline fascia has been established the patient is asked to perform a task that results in activation of the muscles that attach into the fascia (RA, EO, IO and TrA) and/or produce an increase in IAP (head lift, straining, cough, sneeze, active straight or modified leg raise). Clinical experience suggests that a normal response is one in which the tension in the fascia is increased, and the bellies of RA are drawn together (**Fig. 3.9a, b**). Conversely, an abnormal response

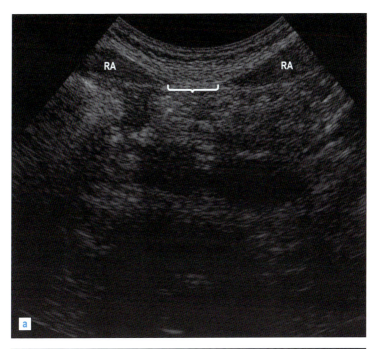

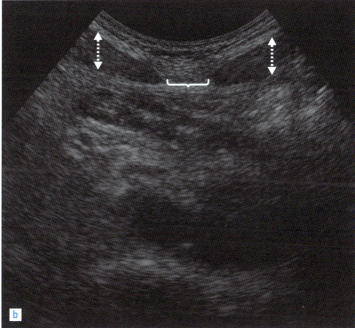

Figure 3.9 USI of the midline abdominal fascia (linea alba) – rectus abdominis (RA) contraction. **a.** Resting transverse ultrasound image of the midline abdominal fascia (bracket). **b.** Transverse image of the midline abdominal fascia at the height of a RA (head lift) contraction. Note the decrease in width of the midline fascia as the two heads of the rectus abdominis are brought together, as well as the increase (dotted arrows) in RA depth as they contract.

is one in which there is either no change or an increase in the distance between the medial edges of RA. A qualitative judgment regarding the movement of the RA bellies with respect to each other or, the change in the width of the midline abdominal fascia (increased, decreased or remained the same) during these events can be made. Beyond this, the width of the fascia can be measured (see Chapter 4) at rest and then again at the height of the event.

Rath et al (1996) studied the width of the linea alba in 40 fresh cadavers, using computerized tomography, in an attempt to establish criteria for the definition of diastasis in two age groups (<45 yrs and >45 yrs). In the younger group a separation >1 cm above the umbilicus, 2.7 cm at the level of the umbilicus and 0.9 cm below became the benchmark, while in the older group the corresponding values were 1.5 cm, 2.7 cm and 1.4 cm. Based on clinical observation Sapsford et al (1998) state that above the umbilicus the width of the linea alba should be between 1 and 2 cm, while below it tends to be narrower.

The linea alba of a nulliparous, non-obese female is seen in the ultrasound image in **Fig. 3.10a**. The medial edges of the RA muscle come together and resemble 'cat eyes' and the layers of the midline fascia are discernible (refer back to **Fig. 2.5b**). This is in contrast to the linea alba of a multiparous, non-obese female (**Fig. 3.10b**) in which there is an obvious increase in width, and slight loss of fascial delineation. These two images represent the range of diversity that can be found in individuals whose myofascial system is capable of generating and distributing tension in a functional manner. Abnormalities include either structural (loss of fascial architecture which allows for a separation >2 cm between the medial edges of the RA) (**Fig. 3.10b**) and/or functional (either an increase or no change in length of the midline fascia with an increase in IAP or muscle activation) factors which point to poor transmission of the tension developed within the muscular system.

If an increase in width or a loss of structural integrity is identified, it is important to consider that clinical management must initially be aimed at improving (use of external support such as a sacroiliac belt or binder) or restoring this structural deficit. Although there has been some indication that rehabilitation may play a role in closing a diastasis (Sheppard 1996), the degree of architectural loss, and the need for a multi-professional (surgical) approach must be considered (Toranto 1990).

LUMBAR MULTIFIDUS

Clinically, there are three main goals associated with imaging of lumbar multifidus. The first is related to resting state, the next

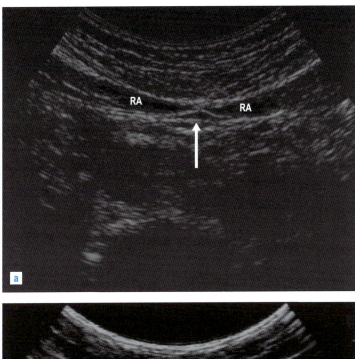

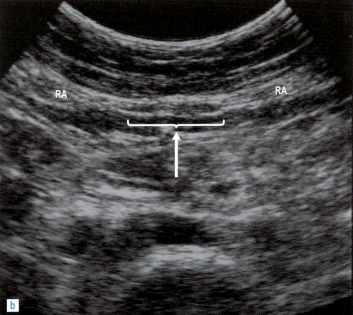

Figure 3.10 USI of the midline abdominal fascia (linea alba). **a.** Transverse ultrasound image of the midline (arrow) abdominal fascia of a non-obese, nulliparous middle-aged female. **b.** Ultrasound image demonstrating an increase in length of the midline (arrow) abdominal fascia in a non-obese, multiparous middle-aged female. Note the increase in distance (parenthesis) between the two heads of RA due to an increase in length of the intervening fascia, as well as the increase in echogenicity of the muscle itself.

considers automatic activation, and the third is dependent upon voluntary effort.

1. Speculate on the resting state (tissue quality), shape and symmetry in size of the lumbar multifidus within the medial compartment of the lumbar fascia.

2. Determine if the lumbar multifidus demonstrates sustained tonic activity during a task that loads the spine and pelvis, such as a side or prone leg lift, and then fully relaxes after the challenge.

3. Determine if the segmental fibres of lumbar multifidus (dMF) can be preferentially activated. Specifically, contracted in relative isolation from the superficial fibres and maintained as an isometric, low-intensity contraction which results in fascial tensioning and co-contraction of other local system muscles (PFM, diaphragm and TrA).

Both the sagittal and transverse imaging techniques outlined in Chapter 2 will be employed to gather this information. The specific indications and limitations for each are outlined below.

Resting state

The literature suggests that the cross-sectional area (transverse plane) of lumbar multifidus in normal young adults should be symmetrical bilaterally at a given segmental level, characteristically oval in shape (Hides et al 1992, 1994), and increase in bulk progressively from L2 caudally to S1 (Amonoo-Kuofi 1983). Stokes et al (2005) investigated these qualities in a large and diverse cohort and confirmed the expectation of symmetry of size within a segment. They identified that although there is individual variation in the transverse plane resting shape of the lumbar multifidus it can generally be categorized as round, oval, or triangular. Furthermore, they speculated that it is the increasing bulk of the muscle that determines this shape. Specifically, as the muscle increases in size it transforms from a round, to oval, to triangular shape, due to the fact that both the medial and anterior confines of the muscle are bony (spinous process and lamina respectively) leaving only the superolateral direction for hypertrophy (which results in a characteristic triangular shape).

Hides et al (1994) employed USI to identify both an alteration in shape (rounder), and decrease in size, of lumbar multifidus ipsilateral and at the level of symptoms in individuals with acute and subacute LBP. They speculated that the rounder shape may have been indicative of hypertonicity; however, this was never formally investigated. The wasting identified by these investigators was detected through cross-sectional area, depth and width measurements of the medial compartment of the lumbar fascia from still transverse plane images (**Fig. 2.9a, b**). The specifics for establishing accurate measurements of this muscle will be considered in greater detail in Chapter 4; however, as the wasting did not spontaneously recover with the resolution of pain, that is, it did not correlate with symptoms (e.g. wasting can be present without pain), there is a basis for contemplating and comparing both the symmetry in size and shape of lumbar multifidus (in a transverse plane) (**Figs 2.8, 2.9a, b**) in a resting state, at various segmental levels prior to further testing.

After commenting on the resting shape and symmetry of multifidus the quality of the muscle tissue should be considered. It is accepted that a decrease in water content in conjunction with an increase in fatty and fibrous content, which can occur with ageing, chronic dysfunction (Tsubahara et al 1995, Campbell et al 2005) and denervation as a result of injury (Andary et al 1998), will result in greater echogenicity of a muscle (that is it will appear more 'white') (Kader et al 2000, Strobel et al 2005). This has been reported in the findings of Stokes et al (2005) who identified an increase in the echoic nature of the multifidus in some of their older subjects. Strobel et al (2005) prospectively evaluated the accuracy of USI in depicting fatty atrophy of the supraspinatus and infraspinatus muscles, with magnetic resonance imaging (MRI) as a reference standard. They proposed a qualitative evaluation tool based upon both the degree of demarcation of architectural characteristics (visibility of muscle contour, pennate pattern, the central tendon), and muscle echogenicity at a set level of gain. On the basis of their findings they concluded that USI is moderately accurate in the detection of significant levels of fatty atrophy in these muscles. Specifically, a three-point scale was used to evaluate the visibility of muscle contours, pennate pattern (architecture of the muscle fibres) and the central tendon (0 = clearly visible muscle contours, fibres and central tendon, 1 = partially visible structures, 2 = structures no longer visible), while a second scale was used to evaluate the echogenicity of the muscle (0 = iso- or hypoechoic in comparison with a reference muscle, 1 = slightly more echoic than a reference muscle, 2 = markedly more echoic than a reference muscle). The reference muscle used was the deltoid, and the diagnosis of fatty atrophy was made with a score of 2 on at least one of the two scales. In keeping with this proposed qualitative analysis the above factors (employing a transverse view which will bring longissimus into the field of view so that it can be used as a reference) can be considered, and commented upon (while maintaining a standard gain setting), while appraising the resting state of multifidus (or for that matter TrA, IO, EO or rectus abdominis).

Tonic activity with spinal loading

After considering the side-to-side symmetry in shape and size of the lumbar multifidus, the patient is asked to perform a task that loads the spine such as an arm or leg lift (prone or side lie) (**Fig. 3.11a, b**). Although there has been some recent disparity regarding locomotion (Saunders et al 2004), current evidence suggests that the deeper segmental fibres of lumbar multifidus (dMF) should contract prior to their more superficial fibres and the thoracolumbar

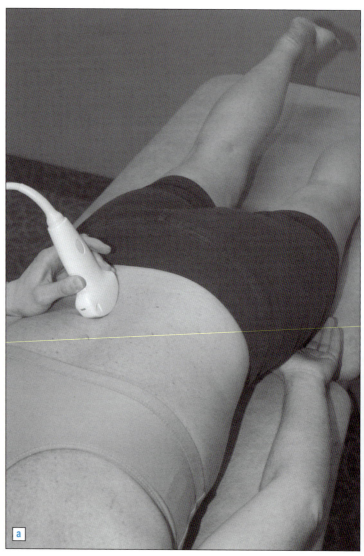

Figure 3.11 Ultrasound probe placement to monitor the lumbar multifidus during **a.** a prone leg lift.

extensors, and remain active in a tonic fashion throughout such a task (Moseley et al 2002). In contrast, delayed and absent activity of dMF has been reported in individuals with LBP (MacDonald et al 2004). Although the pre-activation of dMF is a matter of milliseconds, hence imperceptible to the naked eye, the tonic activity of the entire multifidus muscle during such a task is visible with USI.

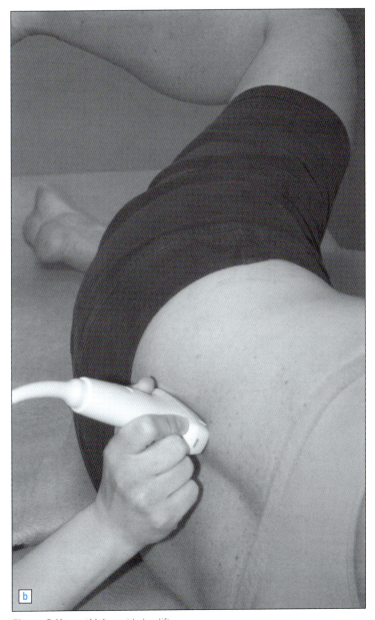

Figure 3.11, cont'd b. a side leg lift.

When limb motion is initiated, a bilateral contraction of both lumbar multifidus and the thoracolumbar extensors should be observed. This will be reflected in a sagittal image by a controlled increase in depth of multifidus and consequential anterior motion of the lumbar vertebral column (**Fig. 3.13b**). The contraction of multifidus should persist during the entire task and then fully relax on completion. Absence, observable delay or premature loss (e.g. relaxation before the leg is lowered) of these architectural changes, or an excessive response (substantial anterior motion of the vertebral) followed by an inability to fully relax after the task are considered abnormal. The first three scenarios indicate a deficiency in either motor control or capacity of the multifidus (or its fascia) and the fourth, potential hyperactivity of either the multifidus or thoracolumbar extensors.

As indicated earlier, RTUS applications that involve limb motion require diligent attention to steady the position, orientation and inward pressure of the ultrasound probe. Failure to do so will result in motion of the probe with respect to the body and false conclusions with regard to muscle behaviour (Pranathi Reddy et al 2001, Whittaker 2004a). In an attempt to control motion and maintain consistent inward pressure of the probe (by matching the outward increase in pressure during the task) the examiner should employ both hands, as well as firmly steady their forearms on the patient's torso and the treatment table.

Preferential activation of the deep segmental fibres of lumbar multifidus

After commenting on the resting state and monitoring the involuntary activity of the entire lumbar multifidus with a task that loads the spine, the patient is asked to produce a voluntary, relatively isolated, contraction of the dMF using one of a variety of verbal commands. Again it is important to acknowledge the lack of evidence suggesting that an inability to achieve this voluntary task is in any way related to the altered involuntary motor control identified in the literature with regard to individuals with LBP. As indicated earlier, the rationale for assessing the ability to produce an isolated voluntary contraction is based upon the evidence indicating that the deep segmental stabilizing muscles are anticipatory and non-direction-specific in their activation (Constantinou & Govan 1982, Hodges & Richardson 1997, Hodges & Gandevia 2000a, Hodges et al 2002, Moseley et al 2002). This anticipatory characteristic suggests that the deep local system muscles have a separate, yet coordinated, control mechanism from that of the superficial musculature. Furthermore, its existence in health, and loss in dysfunction (Richardson et al 2004), necessitates consideration of motor control. Clinically, this involves the evaluation of the ability to access the specific neurological pathways and produce a voluntary isolated contraction of dMF in the absence of superficial fibre activity which can be maintained as an isometric, low-level contraction which results in fascial tensioning and co-contraction of the other local system muscles.

Isolated motor control of the dMF is most easily observed in a sagittal plane (**Figs 2.6, 2.7a, b**). It is important to reiterate that preferential activation evaluates many factors beyond the health of the motor control pathways. For instance the individual's ability and motivation to learn, as well as the ability of the therapist to instruct, will have an influence on the success of this task (Hodges 2005a). Hence, there is no magical cue that will elicit the correct contraction. Some common clinical cues used to elicit a contraction of the dMF include (adapted from Lee 2004):

- 'Imagine that your pelvis is a chicken on a spit. Think about generating a force which would slowly and gently spin it forward'.

- 'Imagine a wire connecting the tip of your tailbone to the back of your head. Think about generating a force which would draw these two points together'.

- 'Imagine a wire connecting your hip bones posteriorly (posterior superior iliac spines) from the left to right side. Think about generating a force which would draw these two bones together'.

- 'Imagine a wire connecting your inner thigh (or pubic bone) to your low back. Think about generating a force which would draw these two points together'.

- 'Slowly and gently draw your lower abdominal wall in towards your spine'.

- 'Slowly and gently think about closing your rear passage (anus)'.

Definition of an isolated dMF contraction

An isolated contraction of the dMF results in a slow increase in depth of the deeper portion (segmental fibres) of the muscle with gradual ventral motion of the lumbosacral vertebral column (detected as inferior motion with respect to the screen) at the segmental levels under investigation (**Fig. 3.12a, b**). The ventral motion of the vertebral column is relative due to the increased depth of the segmental fibres and the stationary position of the probe on the display. The therapist must be vigilant in detecting where the increase in muscle depth occurs (deep vs. superficial)

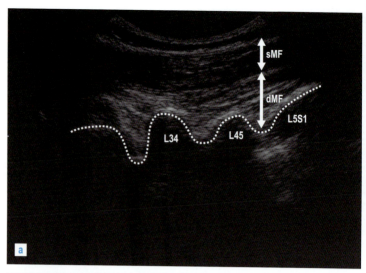

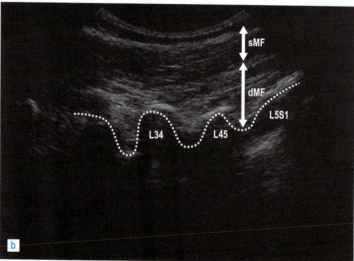

Figure 3.12 USI of the lumbar multifidus (sagittal) – preferential activation. **a.** Resting ultrasound image. **b.** An isolated response of the dMF at L5; note the isolated increase in depth of the deeper fibres, and the anterior movement of the vertebral column at L5.

during the effort as contraction of both the superficial and deep fibres will increase the overall thickness of the muscle; however, only a deep contraction is the ideal response. If the patient is capable of producing an isolated contraction without concurrent superficial muscle activity, then they are asked to repeat the contraction and hold it while they breathe normally. Concurrently, the examiner palpates for a co-contraction of the TrA (**Fig. 3.8**). This will establish the endurance capacity of the dMF, as well as its ability to coordinate and co-contract with the other muscles of the local system.

Abnormal responses

As the response can be segmental, multi-segmental or asymmetrical (Hides et al 1994), imaging should be repeated at various levels bilaterally. Abnormal responses include absent or insufficient recruitment (hypoactivity) of dMF with or without substitution of the superficial muscles (superficial fibres of multifidus, thoracolumbar extensors), or an inability to contract dMF in relative isolation. An

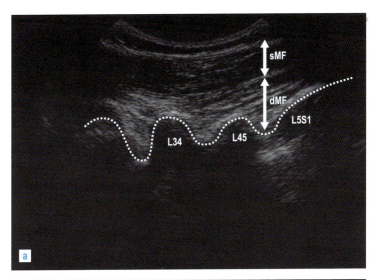

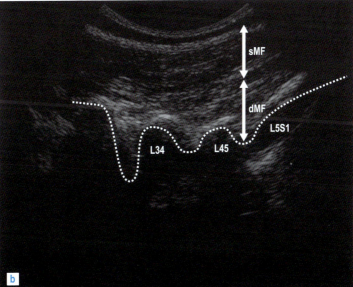

Figure 3.13 USI of the lumbar multifidus (sagittal) – excessive response.
a. Resting ultrasound image **b.** Hyperactive response from the superficial extensors of the lumbar spine; note the increase in depth of the superficial fibres of multifidus (sMF) and the substantial anterior movement of the vertebral column at multiple segmental levels.

absent or insufficient response results in ineffective force closure of the lumbopelvic region secondary to a deficiency in the contractile component (absent or hypoactive contraction, altered length tension or atrophy), and/or a loss of integrity of the fascial system (loss of ligamentous or fascial integrity) (Lee 2004). Furthermore, if the contractile component is incompetent (either due to inadequate activity or bulk), the lumbar fascia surrounding the muscle will not be sufficiently tensioned, and little change will be seen between resting and contracted images.

Co-contraction of both the deep and superficial fibres of multifidus (as well as the thoracolumbar extensors) may result in inappropriate (excessive) force closure of the thorax, lumbar spine and pelvis (Lee 2004). The resultant ultrasound image will demonstrate a concurrent, phasic increase in depth of the entire muscle from the subcutaneous interface to the articular pillar (**Fig. 3.13a, b**) and spinal extension will occur.

When USI is used to assess the behaviour of a muscle there is a tendency to focus all attention upon the display screen. It is critical that the therapist remember that USI is only an adjunct to the examination process, and not abandon other tools such as

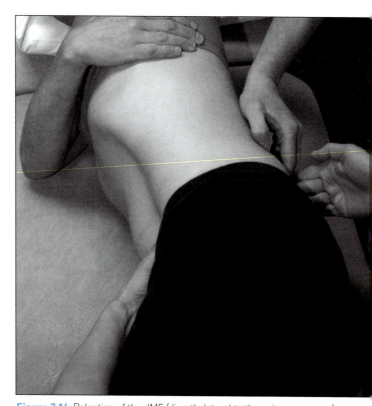

Figure 3.14 Palpation of the dMF (directly lateral to the spinous process).

observation and palpation. It is critical that the patient is observed and dMF is palpated throughout the USI assessment (**Fig. 3.14**). **Tables 3.3** and **3.4** summarize some common observation and palpation considerations and their potential implications.

TABLE 3.3 OBSERVATIONAL CONSIDERATIONS DURING PREFERENTIAL ACTIVATION OF THE DEEP SEGMENTAL FIBRES OF LUMBAR MULTIFIDUS

PHASE	CONSIDERATION	POTENTIAL IMPLICATION
Resting position	Position of the spine (neutral, flexed, extended)	Resting superficial muscle tone
	Symmetry and location of breathing pattern (apical, lateral costal, abdominal)	Degree of abdominal laxity and thoracic elasticity (joint dysfunction, muscle hypertonicity, disease process)
	Movement of the thoracolumbar junction with respiration	Superficial muscle activity
	Resting thoracolumbar lordosis	Resting tone of the thoracolumbar erector spinae
	Asymmetry of paravertebral muscles	Atrophy or hypertonicity
	Scars	Anatomical disruption
During contraction	Movement of the spine (thoracolumbar or lumbar extension, side flexion, rotation etc.)	Superficial muscle activity
	Movement of the rib cage (expansion, clamping down, gripping, symmetry)	Superficial muscle activity
	Visible contraction of the superficial multifidus or thoracolumbar erector spinae	Superficial muscle activity
	Alteration in breathing pattern (holding, valsalva, bearing down)	Superficial muscle activity, underlying breathing dysfunction
	Speed of contraction (phasic vs. tonic)	Type of muscle activated (phasic = superficial)
During relaxation	Inability to fully relax the multifidus and paravertebral muscles	Hypertonicity
	Speed and coordination of relaxation	State of motor control
	Movement of the spine	Relaxation of superficial muscle activity

BLADDER AND PELVIC FLOOR MUSCLES

Clinically, there are three goals associated with imaging of the bladder and PFM. The first is related to resting state, the next

TABLE 3.4 PALPATORY CONSIDERATIONS DURING PREFERENTIAL ACTIVATION OF THE DEEP SEGMENTAL FIBRES OF LUMBAR MULTIFIDUS

PHASE	CONSIDERATION	POTENTIAL IMPLICATION
Resting position	Quality of resting muscle tone (abdominals, paravertebrals etc.)	Resting muscle tone
	Segmental deficit in the bulk of multifidus	Segmental atrophy
	Motion of the thoracolumbar junction with breathing	Superficial muscle activity, underlying breathing dysfunction
	Freedom of the rib cage to disassociate from the pelvis (resistance to rib cage wiggle)	Degree of resting muscle tone
During contraction	Quality of the tension developed with the contraction (slow deep swelling)	Isolated dMF activity
	Quality of the tension developed with the contraction (quick twitch)	Superficial multifidus activity
	Movement of the thoracolumbar junction or rib cage	Superficial muscle activity
	Movement of the pelvis (feel for posterior or anterior tilt)	Superficial muscle activity
	Palpable co-contraction of TrA	Local system co-contraction
	Co-contraction of the oblique abdominals, erector spinae, external rotators of the hip etc.	Superficial muscle activity
During relaxation	Inability to relax the multifidus or paravertebral muscles.	Hypertonicity
	Speed and coordination of relaxation	State of motor control
	Movement of the spine	Relaxation of superficial muscle activity
	Movement of the pelvis	Relaxation of superficial muscle activity

considers automatic activation, and the third is dependent upon voluntary effort:

1. Speculate on the resting state of the PFM, relative position of the bladder, and integrity of the endopelvic fascia.

2. Determine if the PFM demonstrate sustained tonic activity during a task that loads the spine and pelvis such as an ASLR, and then fully relax after the challenge. Furthermore, determine the impact of activities that increase IAP, such as straining, coughing or sneezing, on bladder position.

3. Determine if the PFM (pubococcygeus and iliococcygeus) can be preferentially activated. Specifically, contracted in relative isolation from other muscles (superficial abdominal, gluteal, external rotators and adductors of the hip) and maintained as an isometric, low-intensity contraction which results in fascial tensioning and co-contraction of other local system muscles (dMF, diaphragm and TrA).

Both the sagittal and transverse abdominal imaging techniques outlined in Chapter 2 will be employed to gather this information. The specific indications and limitations for each are outlined below.

Resting state

Prior to assessing the impact of spinal loading and a voluntary contraction of the PFM on the bladder, its resting shape from both a sagittal and transverse point of view should be considered. Every bladder has a unique profile; however, they are typically symmetrical in depth from right to left, and slightly larger in their cranial aspect when moderately full (Walz & Bertermann 1990) (**Figs 3.19a, 3.20a**). Deviations from normal, particularly in the right-to-left symmetry (best viewed in the transverse plane), as well as the resting height of the pelvic floor (best viewed in the sagittal plane), are commonly seen clinically (**Figs 3.15a, b, c, 3.16b, 3.21**). Three of the possible sources of this asymmetry are: resting unilateral hypertonicity (of either the PFMs or oblique abdominals), a loss of integrity of the paravaginal portion of the endopelvic fascia (Ostrzenski & Osborne 1998, Martan et al 2002), and resting unilateral hypotonicity of the PFM (**Fig. 3.15a, b, c**). From the perspective of a still image all three present similarly. Consequently, the source of the asymmetry can only be hypothesized once the impact of an isolated contraction and attempted relaxation on the resting image is considered in conjunction with all other assessment findings.

If the asymmetry is exclusively due to unilateral hypertonicity of either the PFM or abdominal obliques (**Fig. 3.15a**), attempts at an isolated contraction will likely amplify the asymmetry, and be followed by an inability to fully relax. Accompanying clinical signs of hypertonicity may also be present. With respect to the PFM these include an inability to fully empty the bladder during voiding, perineal pain at rest, during intercourse and on contraction, perineal trigger points and intolerance to additional compression to the inferior aspect of the pelvis (FitzGerald & Kotarinos 2003a, Sapsford 2004, Lee 2004). Signs of oblique abdominal hypertonicity include decreased excursion of the lower aspect of the ipsilateral rib cage with inspiration, chest and thoracolumbar pain in sustained

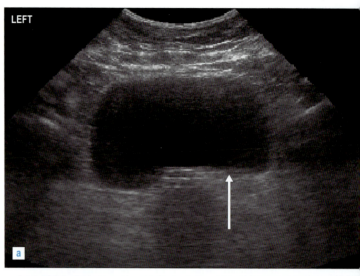

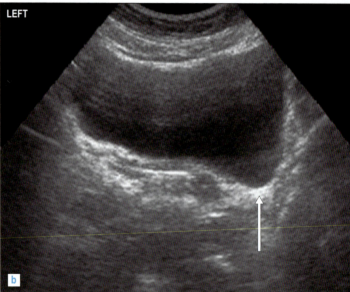

Figure 3.15 USI of the bladder (transverse) – resting asymmetrical presentations. **a.** Hypertonicity of the right side of the pelvic floor (white arrow). **b.** Right paravaginal defect.

postures, abdominal trigger points and intolerance to additional compression of the thorax (Lee 2003). In contrast, if the asymmetry is purely due to a paravaginal defect (PVD) (**Fig. 3.15b**) attempts at either an isolated contraction or voluntary valsalva will amplify the asymmetry. In the case of the isolated contraction the tension of the PFM contraction will not be transmitted to and lift the side of the bladder that has lost its direct fascial support, while with a valsalva the increasing IAP will drive the bladder down into the

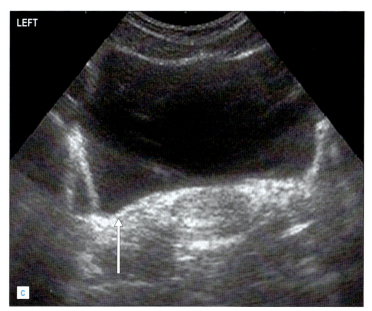

Figure 3.15, cont'd c. Hypotonic left pelvic floor.

slack or deficient fascial gap (Dietz et al 2005). Concurrently, clinical signs consistent with a loss of myofascial support may be present, including: stress and/or urge urinary incontinence, organ prolapse, loss of segmental stability of the ipsilateral sacroiliac joint and an affinity towards additional compression to the inferior aspect of the pelvis (Sapsford 2004, Lee 2004). Moreover, if the asymmetry is due to unilateral hypoactivity of the PFM, attempts at an isolated contraction may begin to normalize the asymmetry and the clinical pattern of presentation will be similar to that of a PVD, indicating a loss of myofascial support (**Fig. 3.15c**).

Diligent observation and clinical reasoning are essential in establishing the source of the asymmetry in order to determine the appropriate intervention and provide an indication of prognosis. If the source of the asymmetry is hypertonicity, treatment will be contrary to that prescribed for asymmetry resulting from hypoactivity. If a structural deficit in the endopelvic fascia is detected, this may suggest a poorer prognosis and the need for possible surgical consultation. To complicate matters further, it is common from a clinical perspective to see combinations of hypertonicity and loss of fascial support. Furthermore, encroachment resulting from a fibroid, cyst or, asymmetry from altered fascial tension as a consequence of surgery must also be taken into consideration.

It is important to consider that the diagnosis of a PVD, fibroid or cyst via an imaging study is a challenging, and in the case of the PVD controversial, undertaking (Nguyen et al 2000, Dietz et al 2005). Furthermore, such conclusions are beyond the scope of

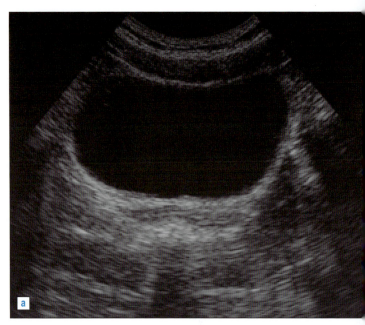

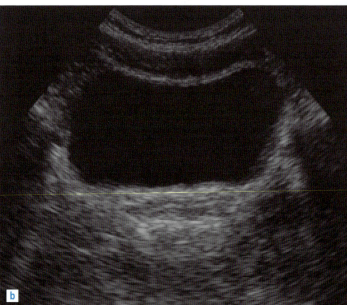

Figure 3.16 USI of the bladder (transverse) – resting symmetrical presentation.
a. Normal resting ultrasound image of the bladder. **b.** Resting image
demonstrating bilateral hypertonicity of the PFM. Note the elevation of the
midline aspect of the inferior border of the bladder.

practice of rehabilitation professionals. However, therapists must be prepared to handle suspicions of such findings in a timely and professional manner. Specifically, it is suggested that if a questionable structure is identified, an image of it should be saved and then passed on to the referring physician with a note indicating that during an USI assessment aimed at determining the functional status of the PFM the structure was detected. Moreover, as the identification of such structures from an imaging study is beyond the therapist's scope of practice, the physician will need to address the necessity for further investigation. If the structure is identified by the patient, then they should be informed of the steps that the therapist is going to take and asked to return to their physician. If, however, the structure is not identified by the patient it is likely prudent to forward the information to the physician without alarming the patient.

Tonic activity and positional bladder stability during spinal loading

After considering the symmetry in size and shape of the bladder, the patient is asked to perform a task that loads the spine and increases IAP, such as cough, sneeze, ASLR (Mens et al 2001, Lee 2004) or a modified active leg raise (Ferreira et al 2004) (**Fig. 3.17a, b**). The PFM, along with TrA and the diaphragm, form the muscular boundaries of the abdominal cavity and work in a coordinated fashion to produce and control IAP (Hemborg et al 1985, Hodges et al 1997, 2003b). The degree of coordination is reflected by the positional stability of the bladder during the loading situation (cough, sneeze, leg lift etc.). This concept is illustrated by the findings of O'Sullivan et al (2002) who identified a significant descent of the bladder in individuals with sacroiliac joint pain during an ASLR, as opposed to a normal comparison group in which little motion was observed. They hypothesized that in the painful group, an altered motor control strategy, which employed a straining-type activation of the diaphragm and superficial abdominal muscles, resulted in an increased IAP, which ultimately overcame the ability of the pelvic floor (PFM and the associated fascia) to support the bladder, and resulted in its descent. Conversely, in the normal group it appeared as though the PFM were capable of balancing the downward pressure on the bladder, keeping it relatively stable throughout the task. This was likely due to a motor control strategy involving a coordinated contraction of TrA, diaphragm and PFM, which produced a reasonable increase in IAP, and pre-activation followed by coordinated tonic activity of the PFM, which served to directly support the bladder. Similar neuromuscular coordination has also been shown to occur during a cough (Constantinou & Govan 1982, Barbic et al 2003). Although

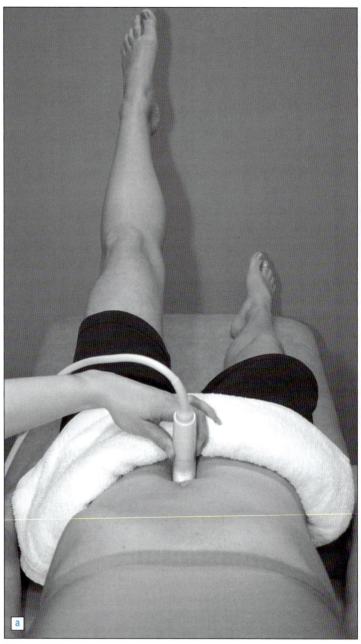

Figure 3.17 Ultrasound probe position to monitor bladder position during
a. an ASLR.

the pre-activation of the PFM is a matter of milliseconds, hence
undetectable to the naked eye, the impact of the coordinated activity of the muscles surrounding the abdominal cavity as well as the
tonic activity of the PFM on bladder position during such tasks is
visible with USI.

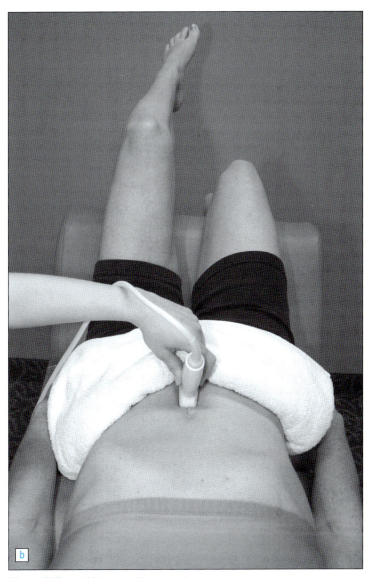

Figure 3.17, cont'd b. a modified leg raise.

During these manoeuvres a sagittal probe position can be used to monitor vertical (descent) motion of the bladder, while a transverse probe position can be employed to observe side-to-side translation. Once the appropriate image has been generated (**Figs 2.11a, 2.13a**) the probe is held still with respect to the abdomen and the patient is asked to cough, sneeze or perform an active straight (or modified) leg raise (**Fig. 3.17a, b**). If there is optimal coordination of the muscles of the region the bladder should remain relatively stationary throughout the task. Several authors have demonstrated that a mild degree of caudodorsal motion of the neck of the bladder occurs with a cough or straining in both standard and patient populations (Meyer et al 1996, Schaer et al 1999, Howard et al 2000) and therefore should be considered normal. A straining or splinting strategy resulting in obvious caudodorsal motion of the bladder on the ultrasound screen from a sagittal view (**Fig. 3.18a**), accompanied by bulging of the lower abdomen (**Fig. 3.18b**), should be considered abnormal and

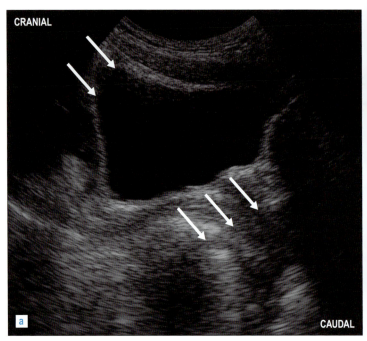

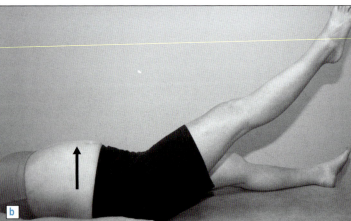

Figure 3.18 Impact of increased IAP and altered PFM function during an ASLR test. **a.** Sagittal image of the bladder depicting caudodorsal motion during an ASLR. **b.** Bulging of the abdomen (arrow) resulting from a straining strategy which leads to a significant increase in IAP during an ASLR.

indicates either a loss of support of the myofascial component of the pelvic floor (a deficiency in either the endopelvic fascia or the motor control and/or capacity of the PFM) and/or an excessive increase in IAP as a result of bracing activation of the diaphragm and abdominal wall muscles (O'Sullivan et al 2002). Alternatively, significant posterior motion of the bladder (detected as inferior motion of the bladder on the ultrasound screen) is also considered non-optimal and although the response may indicate that the excessive increase in IAP, and excessive abdominal wall activation have been met by a contraction of the PFM, it suggests lengthening of the fascia that supports the bladder, which could become problematic with repetition. Furthermore, obvious lateral translation of the bladder (seen in the transverse plane) is also abnormal and may represent either increased contralateral oblique abdominal activity (shifts the bladder away) or insufficient ipsilateral pelvic floor activity (fails to provide support).

As indicated earlier, RTUS applications that involve limb motion require diligent attention to steady the position, orientation and inward pressure of the ultrasound probe. Failure to do so will result in motion of the probe with respect to the body and false conclusions with regard to muscle behaviour and changes in bladder position (Pranathi Reddy et al 2001, Whittaker 2004a). This is particularly important in this circumstance due to the potential for significant increases in IAP and abdominal bulging. Both phenomena have the potential to thrust the probe out of the abdomen, increasing the distance from the probe to the bladder, and produce false motion of the bladder on the display. Consequently, a perineal approach has been advocated as more reliable and valid by several authors (Schaer et al 1999, Pranathi Reddy et al 2001, Thompson et al 2005). In an attempt to control motion and maintain consistent inward pressure of the probe (by matching the outward increase in pressure during the task) the examiner should employ both hands, as well as firmly steady their forearms on the patient's torso and the treatment table.

Preferential activation of the pelvic floor muscles

After observing the resting shape and monitoring the involuntary activity of the PFM during a task that loads the spine and increases IAP, the patient is asked to produce a voluntary, relatively isolated, pelvic floor contraction using one of a variety of verbal commands. As previously mentioned, there is a lack of evidence to suggest that an inability to achieve this task is in anyway related to the altered involuntary motor control identified in the literature with regard to individuals with LBP. However, there is evidence that links an inability to produce an isolated contraction of the PFM with the presence of incontinence (Hay-Smith et al 2001). Clinically, the purpose of the task is to assess the ability to access the specific neurological pathways to these muscles.

It is critical to realize that preferential activation evaluates many factors beyond the health of the motor control pathways. For instance the individual's ability and motivation to learn, as well as the ability of the therapist to instruct, will have an influence on the success of this task (Thompson & O'Sullivan 2003, Hodges 2005a). Hence, there is no magical cue that will elicit the correct contraction. Some common clinical cues include (adapted from Lee 2004):

- 'Slowly and gently contract the muscles in an attempt to slow your flow of urine'.
- 'Slowly and gently drawing your vagina (or testicles) up into your body'.
- 'Slowly and gently think about closing your rear passage (anus)'.
- 'Slowly and gently draw your lower abdominal wall in towards your spine'.

Clinical experience suggests that providing basic guidance about the anatomical location of the PFM in addition to a verbal command is beneficial, as there appears to be a significant number of individuals that confuse their lower abdominal region with their pelvic floor, and a posterior pelvic tilt with a PFM contraction.

Definition of an isolated pelvic floor muscle contraction

The bladder is supported by the PFM and the endopelvic fascia (Aston-Miller et al 2001, Williams 1995). When the midline PFM (pubococcygeus and iliococcygeus) contract they broaden, increase the tension of the endopelvic fascia, and produce encroachment of the bladder wall. This is normally reflected as a slow indentation isolated to the caudodorsal aspect of the bladder wall, accompanied by a cranioventral lift of both the neck and body of the bladder (Bø et al 2001, Christensen et al 1995, Howard et al 2000, Pranathi Reddy et al 2001, Whittaker 2004a) (**Figs 3.19a, b** and **3.20a, b**).

The indentation of the caudodorsal aspect of the bladder wall can be observed in both the sagittal (Bø et al 2003, Thompson & O'Sullivan 2003, Whittaker 2004a, Thompson et al 2005, 2006a) and transverse (Whittaker 2004a, Sherburn et al 2005) planes; however, Christensen et al (1995) suggest that displacement is most easily observed from the sagittal perspective. Clinically, as the response of the PFM is often asymmetrical there is value in screening the contraction from both planes. The sagittal view allows for analysis of cranioventral motion, whereas the transverse view allows for evaluation of the side-to-side symmetry of the contraction. If the patient can demonstrate an isolated contraction of the PFM they

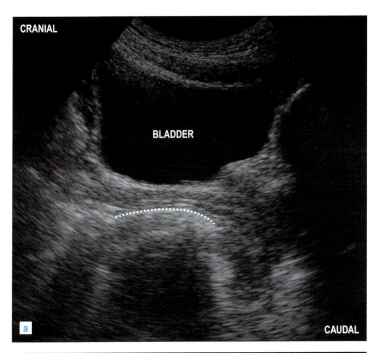

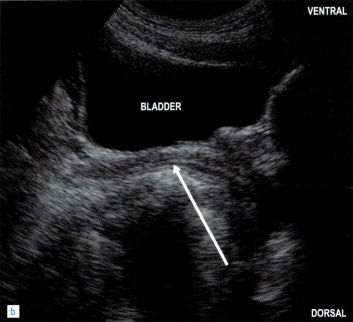

Figure 3.19 USI of the bladder and pelvic floor muscles (sagittal) – preferential activation. **a.** Resting ultrasound image of the bladder, vaginal wall (dotted line) and pelvic floor. **b.** An isolated response of the midline PFM; note the isolated indentation as the vaginal wall is lifted into the caudodorsal aspect of the bladder (arrow).

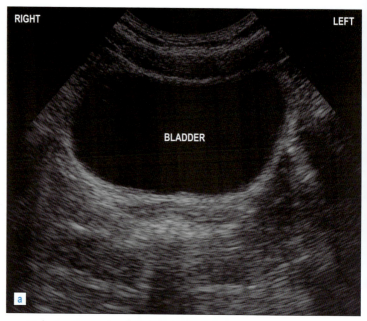

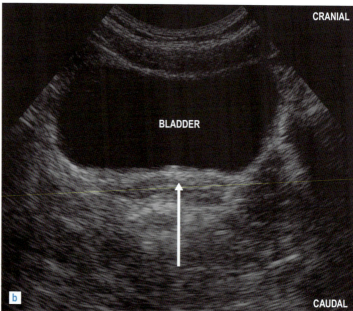

Figure 3.20 USI of the bladder and pelvic floor muscles (transverse) – preferential activation. **a.** Resting ultrasound image of the bladder. **b.** An isolated response of the midline pelvic floor muscles; note the isolated indentation of the caudaldorsal aspect of the bladder (arrow).

are asked to repeat the contraction and hold it while breathing normally. Concurrently, the examiner palpates for a co-contraction of TrA and dMF (**Figs 3.8, 3.14**) (Sapsford & Hodges 2001). This will establish the endurance capacity of the PFM, as well as their ability to coordinate and co-contract with the other muscles of the local system (TrA, dMF and diaphragm).

Abnormal responses

An abnormal response involves absent or insufficient recruitment (hypoactive) of the PFM, with or without excessive activation of the diaphragm, abdominals and external rotators of the hip. Alternatively, the response may result in excessive cranioventral lift, or encroachment of the bladder somewhere other than the caudodorsal wall.

An absent or insufficient response generally indicates ineffective force closure of the lumbopelvic region secondary to a deficiency in the contractile component (absent or hypoactive contraction due to injury, inflammation of adjacent organs, altered length tension, atrophy or impaired nerve supply) and/or a loss of integrity of the fascial system (resulting from birthing trauma, repetitive use of a straining strategy, surgical procedures or genetic disposition) (Lee 2004). Such a response will be identified by an effort that results in negligible encroachment of the bladder wall, or change in the resting image. To complicate matters a similar response will be seen if the bladder is of insufficient volume or, if the PFM are in a state of symmetrical resting hypertonicity (**Fig. 3.16b**), as neither scenario will allow for an observable deformation of the bladder wall or a change in bladder position. An additional consideration is that inappropriate activation of the diaphragm and abdominal wall muscles (either unilaterally or bilaterally) will result in a downward directed increase in IAP, which will not only elevate the resting activity of the PFM, but mechanically hinder elevation of the pelvic floor and the resultant encroachment of the bladder wall (Thompson & O'Sullivan 2003, Thompson et al 2006a). Concluding the response as absent or hypoactive in either of these scenarios would be inaccurate and lead to an inappropriate course of treatment. For example, if the contraction appears absent because the PFM are already in a state of contraction (hypertonicity) and/or being overcome by a large increase in IAP, concluding that there is hypoactivity and then attempting to correct this by encouraging further activation will likely perpetuate the dysfunction, and potentially increase symptoms (FitzGerald & Kotarinos 2003b, Thompson et al 2006b).

If the patient appears to be able to demonstrate an isolated contraction of the PFM it is important to consider the amplitude of the lift, as well as the location of the encroachment of the bladder. Concluding that the myofascial component of the pelvic floor is normal when a successful isolated contraction of the PFM is demonstrated may be erroneous if the lift of the pelvic floor is excessive, or impacts the bladder on its dorsal wall. It is hypothesized that both are indicative of lengthened or incompetent fascial support, and may correlate with a lower resting position of the bladder (**Fig. 3.21a, b**) (Meyer et al 1996). Specifically, if the support system for the bladder is lengthened (either due to birthing trauma or repetitive use of a straining strategy) a PFM contraction will result in greater

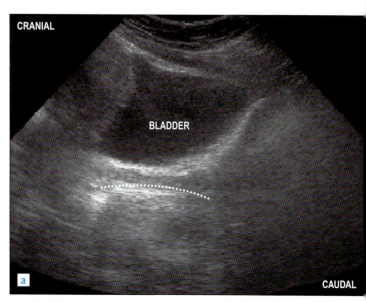

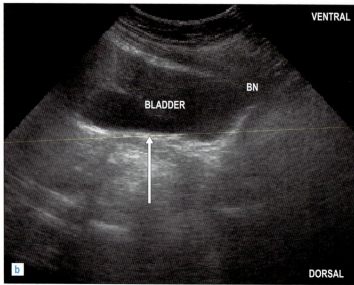

Figure 3.21 USI of the bladder and pelvic floor (sagittal) depicting the impact of a PFM contraction in an individual with incompetent fascia and an altered resting position of the bladder. **a.** Resting ultrasound image of the bladder; note the position of the bladder and its relationship to the vaginal wall (dotted line). **b.** Preferential activation of the midline PFM on an inferior sitting bladder. Note the isolated indentation of the dorsal vs. caudodorsal aspect of the bladder (arrow).

cranioventral displacement of the bladder before the laxity in the fascial system is reeled in (Peschers et al 1996, Bø et al 2003). This concept is further supported by the fact that there are a proportion of individuals that can demonstrate elevation of their pelvic floor when asked, that continue to have symptoms of urinary incontinence (Thompson & O'Sullivan 2003) and pelvic girdle pain (Stuge et al 2006a).

Excessive and concurrent activation of the diaphragm and abdominal wall muscles (e.g. resulting from a splinting or straining strategy) will result in inappropriate (excessive) force closure of the thorax, lumbar spine and pelvis (Lee 2004) and significant increases in IAP (Thompson et al 2006b). The resultant ultrasound image will demonstrate a visible increase in depth of the RA, encroachment of the cranioventral and lateral aspects of the bladder wall, as well as potential concurrent caudodorsal motion of the bladder (**Fig. 3.22a, b**) (Christensen et al 1995, Bø et al 2001). The presence of bladder motion will depend upon whether there is an accompanying contraction of the PFM, which would be identified by either a caudodorsal indentation of the bladder, or preservation of the bladder height as it is thrust posterior. Furthermore, this straining or splinting type of strategy may result in outward pressure of the abdominal wall (which is detectable through the ultrasound probe), and depression of the rib cage or a posterior pelvic tilt may be observed. It is interesting to note that there is a higher prevalence of incontinence and pelvic organ prolapse in individuals that depress their pelvic floor when asked to produce an isolated contraction, which supports the suggestion that chronic use of this motor control strategy leads to damage of the supporting endopelvic fascia (Thompson & O'Sullivan 2003).

FINAL COMMENTS

Although the interpretation of both static and dynamic ultrasound images is a challenging undertaking, the responses observed during each of the preceding imaging applications can be classified into one of three general categories (sufficient, excessive or insufficient) which can then be used to direct treatment (Chapter 5). A sufficient response is one characterized by appropriate force closure of the lumbopelvic region which allows for efficient load transfer, an ability to return to a state of equilibrium, and meets the demands of respiration and continence (Hodges 2005b). That is, a coordinated, isometric co-contraction of the deep muscles, in conjunction with appropriate (dependent on the nature of the task) activation of the superficial muscles, which results in sufficient tension production within the regional fascia allowing for support of the pelvic viscera and skeletal system.

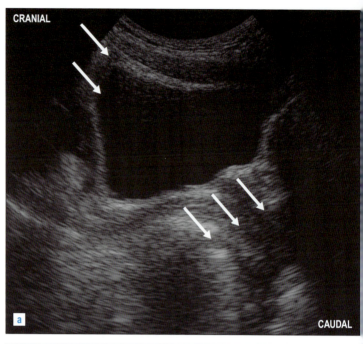

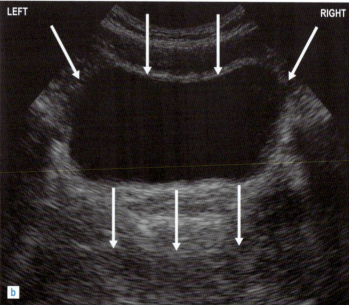

Figure 3.22 USI of the bladder and pelvic floor – excessive response. A representation of the impact of a straining-type strategy on bladder position.
a. Sagittal and **b.** transverse image of the bladder depicting caudodorsal motion of the bladder due to excessive activation of the diaphragm and abdominal wall muscles.

An excessive response is characterized by excessive force closure of the lumbopelvic region due to unwarranted muscle activity which may interfere with load transfer, respiration and/or continence. Symptoms and clinical signs consistent with this type of presentation may coexist and include complaints of chronic tightness, inability to fully void and an intolerance of prolonged positions or weight-bearing situations, as well as the presence of painful trigger points, poor lateral costal expansion of the rib cage with respiration, myofascial restriction of joint motion and an intolerance to further compression through the region (Lee 2004). From a USI perspective an excessive response will present as:

- Inability to relax muscles – a situation in which the muscles of the region are in a state of resting hypertonicity. This may be seen as either respiratory modulation of the abdominal wall, or resting activation of the muscle system.

- Inability to separate the deep and superficial muscles – simultaneous contraction of both the deep and superficial muscles during an attempt at preferential activation (in an attempt to assess its separate control mechanism). It is important to remember, however, that an inability to produce an isolated contraction of a deep muscle may be a result of various factors beyond the health of the motor control pathway, hence should not be considered diagnostic in itself.

- Timing deficit – a situation in which there is either disproportionate excessive activation during, or an observed inability to fully relax a muscle at the completion of, a task such as an ASLR.

An insufficient response is characterized by insufficient force closure of the lumbopelvic region, hence an inability to either effectively transfer load through the region and/or meet the demands of respiration or continence. Symptoms and clinical signs consistent with this type of presentation may coexist and include a feeling of instability, stress or urge urinary incontinence, an intolerance of repetitive loading situations, observable muscle atrophy, observable hernia or abdominal diastasis, positive tests of load transfer and joint stability, as well as an affinity towards further compression through the region (e.g. use of a sacroiliac belt) (Lee 2004). From a USI perspective an insufficient response will present as:

- Hypotonic muscle contraction – a situation in which little or no muscle contraction is detected.

- Incompetent muscle contraction – a situation in which a muscle contraction fails to produce sufficient fascial tension, either due to length–tension issues of the muscle itself or as a result of insufficient muscle bulk within a fascial compartment (e.g. due to insufficient bulk of multifidus within the medial compartment of the lumbar fascia, similar to a lack of sausage meat within a sausage casing, a competent contraction may fail to tension the fascial system).

● Incompetent fascia – a situation in which forces generated from a muscle contraction are not normally distributed due to incompetent fascia (e.g. lengthened linea alba, lengthened linea semilunaris, an abdominal diastasis, or a paravaginal defect of the endopelvic fascia).

● Timing deficiency – a situation in which there is either delayed or inconsistent (premature loss) activation of a muscle during a task such as an ASLR.

Accurate interpretation requires knowledge of the anatomy of the lumbopelvic region as well as motor control concepts concerning postural control, segmental stability, continence and respiration. Beyond this, diligent attention to detail with respect to the ultrasound images themselves, combined with consideration of all the information available from traditional assessment findings (patient history, physical and biomechanical examination) is essential. Ultimately, however, it is continued and thoughtful experience, as well as exposure to ultrasound within a variety of clinical settings, that will improve the confidence and accuracy of the clinician.

4 Image interpretation: quantitative

As indicated in the previous chapter, the use of USI to describe a muscle contraction is a complex issue (Hodges et al 2003a, Hodges 2005a). An encompassing approach suggests a role for both qualitative and quantitative analysis. As the qualitative aspects have been covered, the purpose of this chapter is to provide clinicians with standardized quantitative measurement techniques that are as valid, reliable and potentially reproducible as possible for a *clinical setting*.

A plethora of quantitative measurement techniques aimed at describing the deep muscles of the trunk have been reported in the literature (Houston et al 1994, Schaer et al 1995, Hides et al 1992, 1994, 1995a, Ueki et al 1995, Bø et al 2003, Coldron et al 2003, Hodges et al 2003a, Thompson & O'Sullivan 2003, Bunce et al 2004, Ferreira et al 2004, Stokes et al 2005, Whittaker 2005, Thompson et al 2006b). Generally, the techniques involve the measurement of a static architectural feature (length, width, depth, volume or cross-sectional area) before and after some event (contraction, leg lift, cough, straining or therapeutic intervention). In considering the methodology reported in these studies several important issues arise. Firstly, that accurate measurement is dependent upon the ability of the investigator to consistently generate an image of the structure(s) of interest. Furthermore, that consideration must be given to ensure consistent patient positioning, measurement site, definition of muscle boundaries, as well as probe placement, orientation and inward pressure, during all sets of measurements. Due to the skill and considerable practical experience required to address these issues and employ the technology in a way that generates valid and reliable measurements, either experienced ultrasonographers or investigators that have proven their reliability have been employed in the majority of the studies. This statement is not meant to discourage clinicians from including quantitative measures in their analysis, only to serve as a caveat, particularly to the novice. A clinician cannot expect that they are going to be able to pick up an ultrasound probe for the first time, place it on a patient, and be able to generate accurate and meaningful measurements. However, armed with the information contained within this chapter and the patience to practice and perfect these skills, meaningful clinical measurements are a future possibility.

GENERAL CONSIDERATIONS

With the techniques outlined in this chapter there are reoccurring methodological issues that must be addressed to ensure that the measurements are as accurate and as meaningful as possible. These issues are related to definition of measurement site, definition of muscle borders, and matters related to repeated measurements such as consistent patient positioning, as well as stable probe location, orientation and inward pressure. Furthermore, consideration must be given to the most appropriate method of analysing and reporting the measurements clinically. These topics will be addressed in a general sense, and then specific recommendations with respect to the individual techniques will be outlined below.

Measurement site

When measuring an architectural feature (length, width, depth, volume or cross-sectional area) of a muscle or its influence on an adjacent structure (e.g. bladder), it is critical that the exact site along the length of the muscle, or structure, where measurement is to take place is defined. This is ideally achieved through the use of a bony or fascial landmark within the image which can serve as a standard reference point from which the measurement can be taken at different points in time. Examples include a set distance from the anterior medial fascial attachment of TrA (Whittaker 2005), a set distance from the midpoint of the linea alba, the posterior superior border of the symphysis pubis (Schaer et al 1995) or the posterior border of a vertebral articular process (Hides et al 1995a). Reference points vary depending on the application, and if available, suggestions will be discussed in each of the following sections.

If a consistent reference point is not available within the ultrasound image, then either a carefully defined surface probe location, generic between subjects, or the region of greatest visualized displacement of a structure (e.g. the region of the bladder wall that exhibits the greatest displacement during a PFM contraction) (Thompson & O'Sullivan 2003, Sherburn et al 2005) are options.

However, it is important to note that due to individual anatomical variations and the plasticity of muscle, the standardized surface location or region of greatest displacement will not always correspond to the same point along the length of the muscle or structure between subjects, or within subjects over time.

Definition of borders

Once the measurement site has been defined the examiner must consider how the borders of a muscle are to be designated. The most practical definition is the one provided by Ferreira et al (2004) which identifies the muscle boundary as the edge of the hypoechoic region (the heterogeneous boundary where the pixels transition from dark to light), as opposed to the midpoint of the muscle's fascial delineation (which often varies in thickness). Further, this definition can be extrapolated to other structures such as the bladder wall (Thompson et al 2006a). On a technical note, it is valuable to remember that in situations where it is difficult to identify this transition (e.g. in individuals with hyperechoic muscle layers or, scatter artefact due to a large adipose layer), the gain of the region of interest can be decreased to enhance the delineation of the border (**Fig. 4.1a, b**).

Repeated measurement considerations

If measurements are to be repeated either within or over several sessions, consideration of error due to inconsistent joint or patient position, probe location, probe orientation, or movement of the probe with respect to the body surface must be addressed. Furthermore, attention must be given to ensure consistent inward pressure of the probe as muscle tissue is encapsulated within a fascial sleeve (similar to water in a balloon), and probe pressure can alter its depth and falsely portray a change in architecture.

To eliminate error due to inconsistent joint or patient position several easy steps can be taken. Essentially, all measurements should take place with subjects in a standardized position. Peripheral joint angles can be measured and monitored with a goniometer or, through the use of consistent props such as a bolster or set number of pillows. In an attempt to standardize the angle of spinal joints or the shape of a region of the spine (e.g. lumbar lordosis), a flexible curvilinear engineering ruler can be used to transfer the posture of the region to a trace and vice versa.

With respect to standardizing probe location several unique solutions have been presented in the literature. For instance, palpable anatomical landmarks (inferior border of a spinous process)

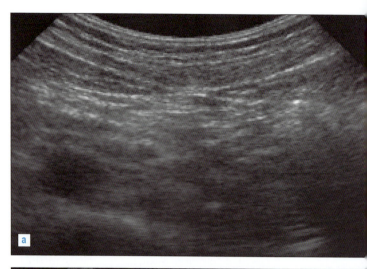

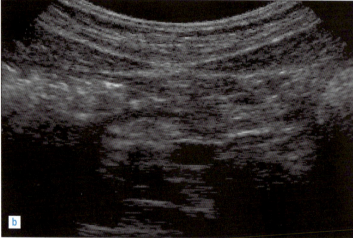

Figure 4.1 Manipulation of gain to accentuate muscle boundaries. **a.** Transverse image of the RA and linea alba (refer to Fig. 2.5 for orientation) with the gain control set at a moderate to high level. **b.** The same image with the total gain decreased. Note how the boundaries of the RA are easier to delineate.

(Hides et al 1995a) or surface markings (moles or scars) can be used. If the time between measurements is short, the location of the probe can be outlined on the skin with a marker. If the time between measurements is longer, then a reusable heavy plastic transparency can be used as a medium on which probe location, unique anatomical marks as well as bony and soft tissue contours can be recorded (Stokes et al 1997, 2005). In an attempt to standardize the probe angle a goniometer can be used to determine the angle of the probe with respect to the surface of the body, or a small construction level can be attached to the probe and the position of the air bubble recorded such that it can be replicated in the future. A unique solution, which may be more appropriate in a laboratory setting, is the use of dense foam, which is strapped to the torso, to house the probe (Bunce et al 2004, Ferreira et al 2004). Regardless of the methodology chosen the imaging hand and forearm should be steadied against the patient's torso and treatment table in preparation to counter any outward pressure imparted to the probe, as well as to prevent movement of the probe with respect to the torso. This is of particular importance in scenarios that involve limb motion or increases in IAP (Pranathi Reddy et al 2001, O'Sullivan et al 2002, Whittaker 2004a).

Beyond these considerations it is critical that multiple trials of a particular measurement are undertaken so that the therapist develops consistency in patient positioning, as well as the placing and handling of the probe. An added step, which would establish that the clinician was capable of using the technology to detect actual change, would be a simple investigation of intra-rater reliability for a specific measurement (Rankin & Stokes 1998).

Analysis and reporting

To further reduce the influence of potential sources of error, measurements should be repeated over several repetitions of the task under investigation and an average value used for analysis (Ueki et al 1995, Coldron et al 2003, Sherburn et al 2005, Whittaker 2005, Ainscough-Potts et al 2006). As a general rule, changes in depth, width, length, cross-sectional area and position should be expressed as either a ratio or a proportion (percentage) of resting depth, width, length, cross-section area or position, as opposed to an absolute value (e.g. millimetres). A ratio or percentage change is useful for comparison between individuals and over time, whereas an absolute value, which is subject to individual characteristics, is not.

MEASUREMENT OF THE LATERAL ABDOMINAL WALL MUSCLES

Of the muscles discussed in this text it is the TrA and IO, along with the PFMs, that have undergone the greatest scrutiny with USI. A review of the literature reveals that the TrA and IO have been measured in a diversity of positions (supine, four-point kneel, sitting and erect) and that various authors report measurements to be valid and reliable (inter and intra) employing an assortment of probes (3.5-5.0 MHz curvilinear to 7-10 MHz linear) and display modes (B or M mode) (DeTroyer et al 1990, Misuri et al 1997, Crichley & Coutts 2002, Kidd et al 2002, Hodges et al 2003a, Bunce et al 2004, McMeeken et al 2004, Ferreira et al 2004,

Henry & Westervelt 2005, Teyhen et al 2005, Whittaker 2005, Ainscough-Potts et al 2006). Consequently, a range of options are available depending on the accessibility of equipment and the specific clinical situation.

Regardless of the parameter measured it is important to remember that there is some debate concerning the correlation between the amount of architectural change seen in the lateral abdominal wall muscles during a contraction, and the quantity of actual muscle activity present (Hodges et al 2003a, McMeeken et al 2004). However, as mentioned in Chapter 3, regardless of the conflicting conclusions regarding the ability of USI to discriminate between moderate and strong contractions (>40% MVC), the two studies to date concur that USI is sensitive to the low-intensity contractions (less than 20-30% MVC) of TrA and IO that are generally being assessed in this text. Both the depth and length measurements described here are appropriate for the clinical setting.

Depth

Numerous methods have been reported for the measurement of the anteroposterior (AP) girth, or depth, of the TrA and IO (DeTroyer et al 1990, Misuri et al 1997, Crichley & Coutts 2002, Kidd et al 2002, Hodges et al 2003a, Bunce et al 2002, 2004, Ferreira et al 2004, McMeeken et al 2004, Teyhen et al 2005, Whittaker 2005, Ainscough-Potts et al 2006, Hides et al 2006). More or less consistent amongst these studies is the use of the anterolateral abdominal wall as the site for measurement. With more in-depth review of the literature it is revealed that several of the studies (DeTroyer 1990, Misuri et al 1997, Crichley & Coutts 2002, Bunce et al 2004, Ainscough-Potts et al 2006, Hides et al 2006) neglect to report the precise point along the length of the muscle where measurement was taken, preferring instead to employ a generic surface probe location, while others (Hodges et al 2003a, Ferreira et al 2004), address this issue with novel methods.

In consideration of these studies, and the logistics of repeatability within a clinical environment, it is suggested that a supine position is employed as it is the easiest in which to reproduce the posture of the thorax, lumbar spine and pelvis, and it is the position in which resting muscle tone is likely to be standardized. The supine position can be modified to crook-lying through the use of a support (bolster) under the legs; however, it is imperative that a consistent device is employed, or that hip and knee flexion angles are recorded, and replicated during repeated measures. With respect to the ultrasound probe it should placed transversely on the abdomen, midway between the iliac crest and the inferior border of the rib cage, on the anterior axillary line, with the medial edge approximately 10 cm from midline (**Fig. 2.2**) (Hodges et al 2003a, Ferreira et al 2004). Once the TrA and IO are identified within the image (**Fig. 2.3a, b**) the medial to lateral placement of the probe is adjusted to ensure that the anterior medial edge of the TrA is approximately 2 cm from the medial edge of the ultrasound image when the subject is relaxed (**Fig. 4.2a, b**). Once a suitable image has been generated it is important to note the specific orientation of the probe. This includes the cranial, caudal, medial and lateral position of the probe, as well as its angle with respect to vertical. Description of probe location and orientation may be facilitated through the use of a transparency trace, goniometer or, a small level attached to the probe.

AP measurements can be made at rest and/or during a contraction depending on the intent of the therapist (e.g. change in resting depth over time, or change in depth during a contraction). If resting images are to be gathered it is important to ensure a state of full relaxation before the image is captured. As the architecture of TrA and IO may alter with respiration every attempt should be made to standardize the point in the respiratory cycle (e.g. at the top of inspiration or at the end of expiration) where the image is collected (Whittaker 2005). If a contracted image is to be gathered it is important to ensure that the image is captured near the height of the contraction. Once the image has been captured, or 'frozen', the internal calipers of the ultrasound unit are used to measure the distance from the most superficial hypoechoic portion to the deepest most hypoechoic portion (**Fig. 4.2a, b**) of the muscle of interest. Either a standard distance from the medial edge of the image or the anterior medial extent of the hypoechoic TrA tissue (**Fig. 4.2a**) can be used as the location to record depth measurements for both the TrA and IO.

In an attempt to improve reliability, the average value of three depth measurements from one image (one at the standardized location, the second 1 cm medial to this site and the third 1 cm lateral) (**Fig. 4.2b**) (Ferreira et al 2004) or a single measurement on three separate images should be used (**Fig. 4.2a**) (Whittaker 2005). To facilitate the comparison of a change in the depth of TrA or IO with some event (contraction, respiration, therapeutic intervention), average values from repeated before and after measures are calculated, and the change is expressed as a percentage of the initial depth.

Length

In a review of the literature only one reference to the measurement of TrA length was identified (Hodges et al 2003a). This parameter was calculated by measuring the change in distance between the edge of the ultrasound image and the most anterior medial extent of TrA before and after a contraction (**Fig. 4.3a, b**). As the

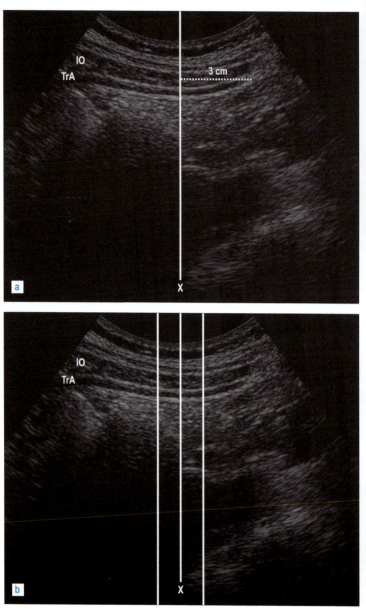

Figure 4.2 Depth measurements of TrA and IO. **a.** A standard line of reference (X) located a set distance (in this case 3 cm) from the anterior medial border of TrA is used as the site at which depth measurements of TrA or IO can be made (adapted from Whittaker 2005). **b.** Additional lines of reference located 1 cm medial and 1 cm lateral to the initial line of reference, upon which repeated measurements can be made (Ferreira et al 2004).

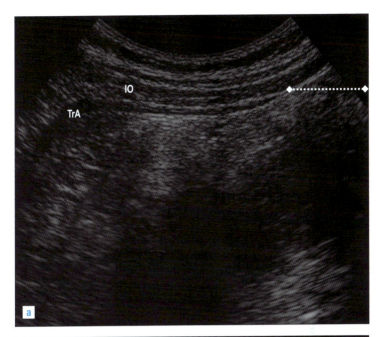

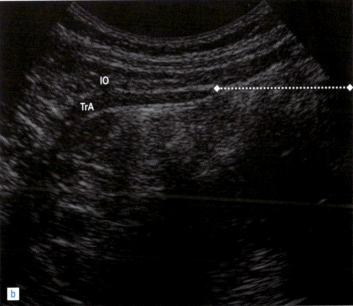

Figure 4.3 Length measurement of TrA. **a.** The internal calipers of the ultrasound unit are used to measure the distance between the anterior medial edge of TrA and the side of the ultrasound image at rest. **b.** This distance increases with an isolated contraction of TrA and represents a decrease in the muscle's length. Consistent probe location during this technique is crucial (Hodges et al 2003a).

posterior insertion of TrA is relatively fixed (although the potential for slack within the lumbar fascia due to atrophy of the muscles contained within its compartments, such as multifidus, has not been investigated), lateral displacement of the anterior medial extent of the muscle reflects a change in its length. As with the depth measurement, all potential sources of error should be considered and minimized, and changes in length reported as a percentage of resting length.

MEASUREMENT OF THE MIDLINE ABDOMINAL FASCIA

Although USI has been used extensively for the assessment of herniation of the abdominal wall (Hodgson & Collins 1991, Rettenbacher et al 2001) a review of the literature revealed only one article alluding to measurement of the midline abdominal fascia (van Uchelen et al 2001). These investigators employed USI to assess the post-surgical status (average of 64 months) of 40 women who had undergone repair of an RA diastasis. Unfortunately, little information was provided with regard to the methodology employed (7.5 MHz linear probe in a supine position), and no reference was made to the validity or reliability of the measurements.

From a clinical perspective there is value in quantifying the width of the midline abdominal fascia at rest, and its change during either an abdominal muscle contraction, an increase in IAP (cough, sneeze, straining, leg lift), or in response to treatment. Again the barriers to reliability lie primarily with accurate and consistent definition of the medial aspect of the RA muscle tissue, as well as reproducibility of probe position, orientation and inward pressure.

Width

The medial to lateral width of the midline abdominal fascia can be determined in a transverse plane (**Fig. 2.4**) (van Uchelen et al 2001, Whittaker 2004b). In consideration of the literature to date and the logistics of repeatability within a clinical environment, it is suggested that a supine position is employed as it is the easiest in which to reproduce the posture of the thorax, lumbar spine and pelvis, and it is the position in which resting muscle tone is likely to be standardized. The supine position can be modified to crook-lying through the use of a support (bolster) under the legs; however, it is imperative that a consistent device is employed, or that hip and knee flexion angles are recorded, and replicated during repeated measures.

As there are no bony landmarks available within the ultrasound image to assist in standardizing the midline transverse probe location, the best option is to measure either down from the inferior border of the xiphoid process or, up from the superior border of the symphysis pubis and mark the skin. The probe can then be placed either directly above or below this mark. Clinically, the umbilicus is a surprisingly mobile structure and not appropriate as a point of reference. Once the medial borders of the RA at the level of interest have been identified (**Fig. 4.4**) the specific orientation of the probe should be noted. This includes the cranial, caudal, medial and lateral position of the probe, as well as its angle with respect to vertical. As mentioned above, this may be facilitated through the use of a transparency trace, goniometer or a small level attached to the probe.

Measurements can be made at rest and/or during an event (contraction or increase in IAP) depending on the intent of the therapist (e.g. change in width over time, or change in width during an event). If resting images are to be gathered it is important to ensure a state of full relaxation before the image is captured. As the midline architecture may alter with respiration it is important to standardize the point in the respiratory cycle (e.g. at the top of inspiration or at the end of expiration) where the image is collected. If a contracted image is to be gathered it is important to ensure that the image is captured near the height of the contraction. Once the image has been captured, or 'frozen', the internal calipers of

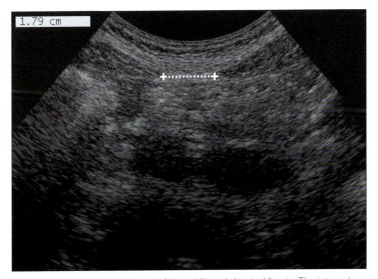

Figure 4.4 Width measurement of the midline abdominal fascia. The internal calipers of the ultrasound unit are used to measure the linear distance (1.79 cm) between the medial most hypoechoic portions of RA (+).

the ultrasound unit are used to measure the distance from the most medial hypoechoic portion of the right RA belly to the medial most hypoechoic portion of the left (**Fig. 4.4**). In an attempt to improve reliability, the average linear value generated from three images, expressed in millimetres, should be used for analysis. To facilitate the comparison of a change in width as the result of some event, average values from repeated before and after measures are calculated and the change is expressed as a percentage of the initial width.

MEASUREMENT OF LUMBAR MULTIFIDUS

An analysis of the literature reveals that measurements of the lumbar multifidus, and erector spinae, have been generated in a variety of planes (sagittal and transverse) as well as positions (prone, side-lie and sitting), and reported to be both valid and reliable (inter and intra) (Hides et al 1992, 1994, 1995a, Coldron et al 2003, Watanabe et al 2004, Stokes et al 2005). Unlike the muscles of the lateral abdominal wall, it is important to acknowledge that the lumbar multifidus is challenging to image, interpret and measure due to the fact that its lateral border with longissimus is often difficult to distinguish, and that there is no obvious fascial delineation between the deep segmental, and superficial multi-segmental fibres. Although both linear (sagittal and transverse planes) and cross-sectional area (transverse plane) measurements are described here the linear techniques are most accessible, require less skill, and consequently are more appropriate for clinical environments. Moreover, in a prospective study of 120 individuals (68 females aged 20-64 and 52 males aged 20-69) Stokes et al (2005) concluded that linear measurements (anteroposterior × mediolateral) correlated highly with cross-sectional area.

Regardless of the plane or parameter measured it is important to note that an increase in the architecture of the lumbar multifidus with an event (contraction, treatment) reflects an increase in depth, width or cross-sectional area of the entire muscle, and is not specific to the deep segmental fibres. It is also important to consider that the anteroposterior dimensions of the multifidus muscle vary considerably within the confines of one vertebral level (e.g. depth at the level of the facet joint is less than over the lamina), and can double between levels (Hides et al 1995a, Stokes et al 2005). Consequently, if a measurement is to be repeated at a later point in time to demonstrate efficacy of a therapeutic intervention it is crucial that the position of the patient, the reference point for measurement, and the angle of the probe are standardized.

Depth

The anteroposterior (AP) girth, or depth of lumbar multifidus, can be determined in either a sagittal or transverse plane, utilizing either a prone or side-lying position (Hides et al 1992, 1994, 1995a, Coldron et al 2003, Stokes et al 2005). In an attempt to standardize joint position for test–retest purposes, as well as to facilitate access to the muscle, the lumbar lordosis is minimized. This entails the use of a pillow under the lower abdomen in prone, and manual positioning with support of any width discrepancy between the hips and waist with a folded towel in side-lying. To ensure that the multifidus at the segmental level of interest is maintained within the ultrasound image, the midpoint (cranial to caudal) of the spinous process at that level can be marked on the patient's skin. This mark can then serve as a visual reference while generating and refining either a sagittal or transverse image (**Figs 2.6, 2.8**). Once a suitable image has been generated (**Figs 2.7a, b, 2.9a, b**) it is important to note the specific orientation of the probe. This includes the cranial, caudal, medial and lateral position of the probe, as well as its angle with respect to vertical.

Measurements can be made at rest and/or during a contraction depending on the intent of the therapist (e.g. change in resting depth over time, or change in depth during a contraction). If a resting image is to be gathered, and a leg lift was employed to differentiate the multifidus from longissimus, it is important to ensure a state of full relaxation, before the image is captured. If a contracted image is to be gathered it is important to ensure that the image is collected near the height of the contraction. Once the image has been frozen, the greatest perpendicular AP (depth) distance from the border of the lumbar fascia with the subcutaneous tissue to either the midpoint of the articular process, or the midpoint of the lamina can be measured with the internal calipers of the ultrasound unit, compared (**Figs 4.5a, b, 4.7a**) and recorded. Again it is critical to indicate if the measurement reflects the depth to the articular process or to the lamina.

A similar (sagittal) procedure can be used to measure the depth of the erector spinae by simply moving the probe further lateral such that the posterior surface of the transverse process is visible within the field of view (Watanabe et al 2004). The perpendicular AP (depth) distance from the border of the lumbar fascia with the subcutaneous tissue to the midpoint of the transverse process can be measured with the internal calipers of the ultrasound unit, compared and recorded (**Fig. 4.6a, b**). It is important to understand that due to the unusual morphology of the lumbar erector spinae musculature the actual muscle being measured at each level may differ. Consequently, knowledge of the sagittal plane anatomy of these muscles is required for interpretation.

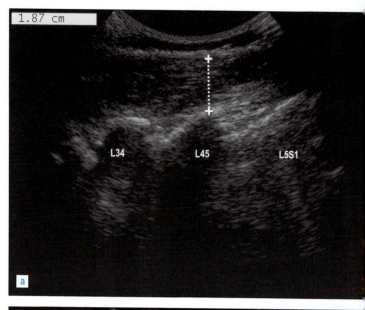

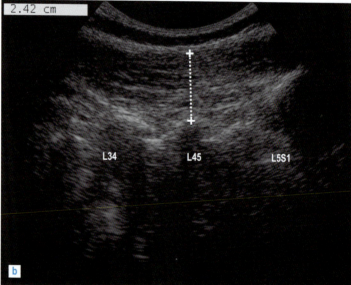

Figure 4.5 Depth measurement of lumbar multifidus (sagittal). The internal calipers of the ultrasound unit have been used to measure the depth of the muscle from its border with the subcutaneous fascia to the posterior aspect of the L45 articular process at **a.** rest (1.87 cm) and **b.** after an isometric contraction (2.42 cm) (Stokes et al 2005).

Once again, to improve reliability, the measure should be repeated and an average linear value used for analysis. To express a change in depth of either the multifidus or erector spinae, average values from repeated before and after measures are calculated and the change is expressed as a percentage of the initial depth.

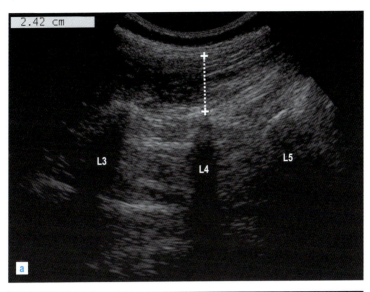

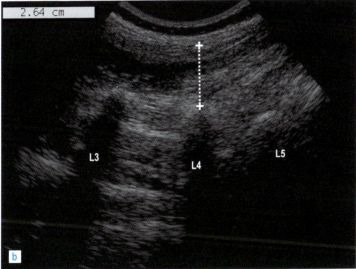

Figure 4.6 Depth measurement of lumbar erector spinae (sagittal). The internal calipers of the ultrasound unit have been used to measure the depth of the muscle from its border with the subcutaneous fascia to the posterior aspect of the L4 transverse process at **a.** rest (2.42cm) and **b.** after an isometric contraction (2.64cm) (Watanabe et al 2004).

Width

The mediolateral (ML) width of lumbar multifidus can be determined in the transverse plane, using either a prone or side-lying position (Hides et al 1992, 1994, 1995a, Coldron et al 2003, Stokes et al 2005). As with the preceding depth measurement, the lumbar lordosis should be minimized and a mark should be placed on the patient's torso at the midpoint (cranial to caudal) of the spinous process of the segment of interest. This mark can then serve as a visual reference, ensuring that the multifidus on the side and at the level of interest is kept within the field of view (**Fig. 2.8**). Multifidus is encapsulated within the medial compartment of the lumbar fascia. This compartment is bound by the spinous process medially, the lamina anteriorly, the fascial layer delineating it from longissimus laterally, and subcutaneous tissue posteriorly. It is relatively easy to discriminate the spinous process, lamina and subcutaneous tissue however, due to the fact that the lateral fascial delineation can lie parallel to the propagating ultrasound wave it is often difficult to distinguish. As the delineation of this lateral border is essential to the accuracy of this measurement, the probe can be tilted slightly lateral so that a greater proportion of the sound beam encounters the fascia at a perpendicular angle. Further Stokes et al (2005) allude to the fact that the fascicular structure of multifidus differs from that of longissimus, and attention to this transition, particularly with a leg lift, can serve as additional assistance. After a suitable image (**Fig. 2.9a, b, Fig. 4.7a, b**) has been generated it is important to note the specific orientation of the probe.

Measurements can be made at rest and/or during a contraction depending on the intent of the therapist (e.g. change in resting width over time, or change in width during a contraction). If a resting image is to be gathered, and a leg lift was employed to differentiate the multifidus from longissimus, it is important to ensure a state of full relaxation before the image is captured. If a contracted image is to be gathered, it is important to ensure that the image is collected near the height of the contraction. Once the image has been frozen, the internal calipers of the ultrasound unit can be used to measure the greatest horizontal ML (width) distance from the lateral aspect of the spinous process to the fascial boundary with longissimus (**Fig. 4.7b**). To improve reliability, the measure should be repeated and an average linear value used for analysis. To express a change in width, average values from repeated before and after measures are calculated and the change is expressed as a percentage of the initial width.

Cross-sectional area/circumference

The cross-sectional area (CSA) of lumbar multifidus can be determined in the transverse plane, utilizing either a prone or side-lying position (Hides et al 1992, 1994, 1995a, Coldron et al 2003, Stokes et al 2005). Clinicians should consider that an accurate CSA measurement of lumbar multifidus requires considerable diligence and

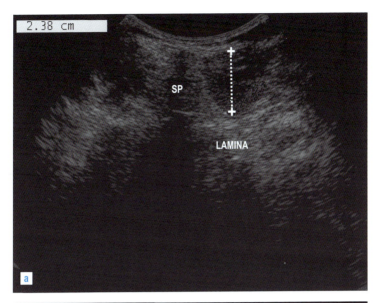

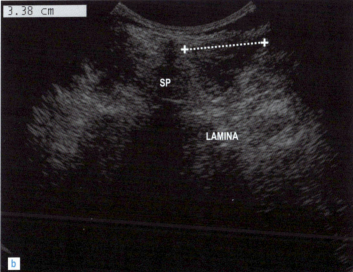

Figure 4.7 Depth and width measurements of lumbar multifidus (transverse). **a.** The internal calipers of the ultrasound unit have been used to measure the greatest depth of multifidus from its border with the subcutaneous fascia to the superior aspect of L4 lamina. **b.** The internal calipers of the ultrasound unit have been utilized to measure the greatest width of multifidus from its medial border with the spinous process to its lateral border with longissimus (Stokes et al 2005).

practical expertise; as such the linear measurements outlined above may better serve their purpose.

As with the preceding measurements the lumbar lordosis should be minimized and the segment of interest can be kept within the field of view by attending to a mark on the patient's torso representing the midpoint (cranial to caudal) of its spinous process (**Fig. 2.8**). As with the width measurement above, the delineation of the lateral border of multifidus is essential to the accuracy of this measurement and the therapist should employ the suggestions outlined. After a suitable image (**Fig. 2.9a, b, Fig. 4.8a, b**) has been generated, the specific orientation of the probe should be noted.

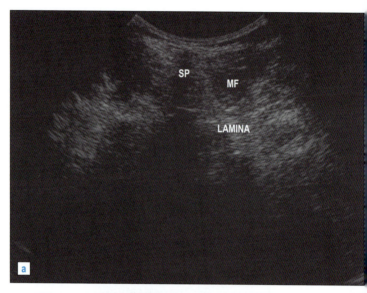

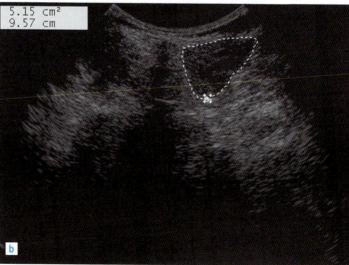

Figure 4.8 Cross-sectional area measurement of lumbar multifidus (transverse). **a.** Transverse image of the right multifidus compartment at the level of L4; SP = spinous process, MF = multifidus. **b.** The internal calipers of the ultrasound unit have been used to trace the circumference (9.57 cm) of the multifidus from which a CSA (5.15 cm²) is estimated.

Measurements can be made at rest and/or during a contraction, depending on the intent of the therapist (e.g. change in resting CSA over time, or change in CSA during a contraction). If a resting image is to be gathered, and a leg lift was employed to differentiate the multifidus from longissimus, it is important to ensure a state of full relaxation before the image is captured. If a contracted image is to be gathered it is important to ensure that the image is collected near the height of the contraction.

Several options exist for calculating CSA and the clinician must choose between tracing around the inner edge of the multifidus border with the internal cursor or using the software applications of the ultrasound unit associated with approximating circumference. For instance, most imaging units have the option of creating the best-fit ellipse either to several points marked on the circumference or to a line representing the diameter of the compartment in question. Once the circumference value has been established, the ultrasound unit calculates a corresponding CSA (cm^2). The most commonly reported method involves tracing the borders of the compartment (**Fig. 4.8a, b**) and although this may be most valid, it does require greater expertise. Regardless of the methodology chosen it is imperative that it is used consistently during testing and in test–retest situations. To improve reliability, the measure should be repeated and an average CSA value used for analysis. To express a change in CSA, average values from repeated before and after measures are calculated and the change is expressed as a percentage of the initial CSA.

MEASUREMENT OF BLADDER WALL MOTION

USI has been used as a valid and reliable (inter and intra) technique to measure the impact of a PFM contraction or an increase in IAP (straining, cough, sneeze or ASLR), on the bladder from a variety of approaches (transperineal and transabdominal) planes (sagittal and transverse) and positions (Wijma et al 1991, Dietz & Clarke 2001, Dietz et al 2001, Pranathi Reddy et al 2001, Peschers et al 2001a, b, Beer-Gabel et al 2002, Murphy et al 2002, O'Sullivan et al 2002, Bø et al 2003, Thompson & O'Sullivan 2003, Thompson et al 2005, 2006a, b). The findings of these studies have been further supported by several magnetic resonance imaging (MRI) investigations (Christensen et al 1995, Fielding et al 1998, Bø et al 2001). Specifically, Christensen et al (1995) employed supine MRI to reveal bladder wall movement during a voluntary PFM contraction in asymptomatic females. They detected that the greatest amount of motion (7.0 ± 2.8 mm) occurred at the gluteal (caudodorsal) region of the bladder wall, and that this displacement was most easily observed from the sagittal plane. Bø et al (2001) recon-firmed the elevating function of the PFM through dynamic MRI in a seated position, and measured the inward movement to be 10.8 ± 6.0 mm in a group consisting of both continent and incontinent women. Furthermore, they demonstrated a mean downward motion of 19.1 ± 7.4 mm associated with straining.

Traditionally, the transperineal approach (placement of the ultra-sound probe in a sagittal plane along the midline of the perineum) has been considered to have superior reliability to the abdominal approach as both the stationary pubic symphysis and the proximal junction of the bladder neck are included within the field of view, and can serve as points of reference. Thompson et al (2005) com-pared sagittal transperineal and transabdominal approaches during a PFM contraction, straining and an abdominal curl in a group of normal women. They concluded that there was a significant cor-relation between the measurements gathered from either approach across the tasks. Furthermore, that the sagittal transabdominal approach was not only reliable, but a non-invasive method of assess-ing bladder motion. Although movement of the gluteal wall of the bladder can be measured in both sagittal and transverse planes, at rest or before and after some event (PFM contraction, cough, sneeze, straining, ASLR), the methodology is similar. The sagittal technique (**Figs 2.10, 2.11a, b**), which is easier to standardize and consequently is more appropriate for clinical environments, is described here (Murphy et al 2002, Bø et al 2003, Thompson & O'Sullivan 2003, Thompson et al 2005, 2006a, b).

In consideration of the literature to date and the logistics of repeatability within a clinical environment, it is suggested that the measurements are gathered with the patient in a supine position as it is the easiest in which to reproduce the posture of the thorax, lumbar spine and pelvis. Furthermore, it is the position in which resting muscle tone is likely to be standardized. The supine position can be modified to crook-lying through the use of a support (bolster) under the legs; however, it is imperative that a consistent device is employed, or that hip and knee flexion angles are recorded, and replicated during repeated measures.

Unique to this measurement application is the influence of volume on bladder mobility. Specifically, Dietz & Wilson (1999) demonstrated increased mobility with smaller bladder volumes. Consequently, every attempt must be made to standardize this parameter. From a research perspective this typically involves com-plete emptying of the bladder followed by the insertion of a catheter and a specific volume of fluid. Clinically, this can be achieved by asking the patient to void approximately one hour prior to the assessment, to then drink 500–600 ml of water and refrain from voiding until after the assessment is completed (Thompson &

O'Sullivan 2003). It is important to indicate to patients that unlike other abdominal ultrasound scans (such as those associated with more traditional imaging goals) where the bladder needs to be near full capacity to serve as an acoustic window, overfilling in this situation will actually interfere with the assessment process.

With respect to ultrasound probe placement a direct midline sagittal approach allowing for a view of the bladder, as much of the neck of the bladder as possible, and the interface between the levator plate and gluteal border of the bladder, is ideal (**Fig. 2.11a**). Once this image has been generated, the specific orientation of the probe should be noted. As there are no bony landmarks available within the ultrasound image to assist in standardizing probe location, it is crucial that surface markers, and the position of the probe from its cranial, caudal, medial and lateral perspective, as well as its angle with respect to vertical, are recorded. As with the previous applications, this may be facilitated through the use of a transparency trace, goniometer or a small level attached to the probe.

Measurements can be made at rest and/or during a contraction, cough, strain or ASLR depending on the intent of the therapist. The methodology involves identifying and measuring the region of the bladder wall that exhibits the greatest displacement during the event. Specifically, a marker is placed on the most mobile region of the bladder wall at rest, and then the individual is asked to perform the task under investigation. At the height of the event the image is frozen and the internal calipers of the ultrasound unit are used to measure the movement of the reference point during the event (**Fig. 4.9a, b**) (Bø et al 2003, O'Sullivan & Thompson 2003, Sherburn et al 2005, Thompson et al 2005, 2006a, b). Although the description of the technique appears somewhat subjective, it has been shown to have both inter- and intra-rater reliability (Murphy et al 2002, Thompson & O'Sullivan 2003). However, it may be possible to improve the objectivity of the method by measuring the distance from the posterior proximal junction of the neck of the bladder (if visible) to the most displaced region of the bladder wall.

A further consideration is that the resultant motion of the bladder wall is oblique in nature and has both a horizontal (anterior or posterior) and a vertical (cranial and caudal) component. However, as the corresponding anatomical planes are not distinguishable within the ultrasound image, it is best to record the angle of the direction of motion from the horizontal border of the ultrasound image. As with previous applications, in an attempt to increase reliability this measurement can be repeated and both the average linear value expressed in millimetres as well as the average angle from image horizontal, used for analysis.

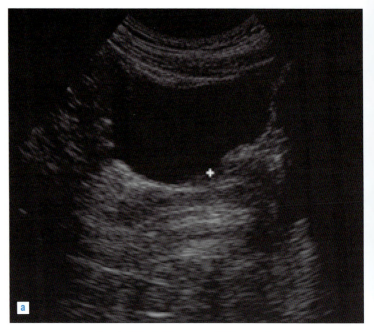

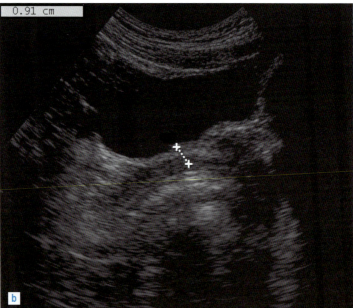

Figure 4.9 The impact of a PFM contraction on the bladder (sagittal).
a. Sagittal image of the bladder at rest. Note the marker (+) on the caudodorsal region of the bladder wall. **b.** The internal calipers of the ultrasound unit are used to measure the movement (0.91 cm) of the region of the bladder wall that corresponds to the marker in the resting image (Thompson & O'Sullivan 2003).

CONCLUSION

The accurate measurement of static ultrasound images is a challenging undertaking. In an attempt to master the skills required, clinicians are encouraged to be as diligent as possible in their methodology, to practice on a variety of body types and, as their skills improve, a variety of postures (seated, standing, four-point kneel etc.). With regard to interpreting the numbers it is critical that they are reported only for what they represent, which is specifically a change in the two-dimensional shape of a muscle or the bladder. As pointed out repeatedly in Chapter 3, a bigger change in muscle architecture, or lift of the bladder, is not always better or ideal, while little or no change in muscle architecture or position of the bladder does not necessarily indicate a lack of muscle activity. To prevent being misled, clinicians should interpret these quantitative measurements alongside the qualitative factors previously outlined and in light of traditional assessment findings.

5 Treatment applications

Conscientious clinicians strive to be as evidence informed in their practice as possible; however, situations arise daily in which the clinical reasoning process leads to the use of techniques, technology or regimes that have yet to withstand scientific scrutiny with regard to their therapeutic utility. Occasionally, this is due to the infancy of the technique, technology or regime. More commonly, however, the procedure is not intended as a stand-alone intervention, hence cannot be studied in a way that meets current scientific scrutiny (Delitto 2005). To confuse matters further, most interventions are appropriate in very specific situations and/or populations (e.g. you would not expect a prescription for antibiotics if you have a fungal infection), and until diligent inquiry to define the situation or specific population that would benefit from the intervention occurs, investigations into its efficacy are often unfavourable in their conclusions. USI has fallen prey to all three of these issues and as a result, evidence supporting its clinical significance is only beginning to emerge (Dietz et al 2001, Kermode 2004, Henry & Westervelt 2005). Hence, the foundation for this chapter is evidence-informed clinical experience and observation.

Clinically, USI has been found to be an invaluable tool in the management of lumbopelvic dysfunction (LPD). As demonstrated in the preceding chapters it complements traditional methods used to assess this region and provides information that has been previously unattainable (e.g. integrity of the abdominal or endopelvic fascia, functional status of the PFM, and the presence or absence of tonic sustained activation of the local system muscles during activities that load the region) but that is crucial to the development of an appropriate rehabilitation strategy. However, the value of USI extends beyond the assessment process, holding value for both the therapist and the patient during the treatment stage. More specifically:

- USI improves the instructional, palpatory and observational skills of therapists that have repeated clinical exposure to it as a means to confirm or negate their findings.

- RTUS is an unrivalled educational tool that allows a therapist to explain and physically demonstrate to a patient the subtleties of their specific motor control impairment.

- RTUS is an invaluable form of biofeedback, and serves as a basis for the provision of knowledge of results, when attempting to either increase or decrease activity of a specific muscle or coordinate activity within muscles of a region (motor learning, motor skill acquisition).

The purpose of this chapter is to provide clinical guidance in the use of USI in the treatment of LPD. However, in shifting the focus from the complementary role that USI has to play in assessment (Chapters 2, 3 and 4) to treatment, a considerable gap in the clinical reasoning process is created. It is critical to understand that the information gathered with USI alone is insufficient to propose a physical diagnosis or course of rehabilitation. Additional information stemming from a detailed history, as well as a thorough physical and biomechanical examination, is required before analysis and intervention can occur. It is beyond the scope of this text to provide an outline for the history, physical and biomechanical examination process, to delve into the intricacies of defining impairment, or to outline a comprehensive programme for rehabilitation of the lumbar spine and pelvis. Nevertheless, such knowledge is crucial if the information gathered with USI is to be exploited to its fullest extent, and integrated appropriately into the rehabilitative process. This information is substantial, and thankfully is covered in comprehensive detail elsewhere (Lee 2004, Richardson et al 2004). There are, however, several fundamental concepts that will be presented here as an attempt is made to clarify under what conditions, and by what means, the use of RTUS can augment treatment.

GENERAL TREATMENT PRINCIPLES

The importance of postural control and in particular, coordinated muscle effort (neuromuscular control), has received considerable attention with respect to the rehabilitation of LPD in recent years (see Lee 2004 and Richardson et al 2004 for a summary). This is due to an accumulation of evidence pointing to altered neuromuscular control (motor control) in individuals with persistent and reoccurring LPD (Deindl et al 1994, Hodges & Richardson 1996, Jull & Richardson 2000, Barbic et al 2003, Hodges & Moseley

2003, Hungerford et al 2003, Richardson et al 2004). Specifically, the altered control tends to present as a loss of anticipatory and non-direction-specific activation of the deep muscles (TrA, dMF, the diaphragm and the PFM) and increased or augmented activation of the superficial muscles in the region (see Hodges & Moseley 2003 for a summary). Further, evidence indicates that these deficits do not consistently recover with the resolution of pain (Hides et al 1994, 2001), and are not addressed with traditional exercise programmes focused on increasing strength and functional capacity (Stuge et al 2006b). The clinical extrapolation of this work is that the initial and pivotal focus in rehabilitation must be to address these motor control alterations. This is achieved by first eliminating any unwarranted activity (hypertonicity) in the superficial muscles of the region, followed by isolated and then coordinated coactivation of the deep trunk muscles, cognitively and as independently as possible from the superficial muscles. Once achieved, the retraining process can proceed with integration of the two muscle systems during an increasingly challenging progression of tasks, ending ultimately with functional movement experiences with specific importance to the patient (Jull & Richardson 2000, Lee 2004, Richardson et al 2004). Throughout each of these phases it is critical to remember that the goal is to train the mechanism that identifies what the demands of each loading situation are, the spectrum of responses that the lumbopelvic region is capable of meeting these demands with, and ultimately the ability to match the appropriate response to the demands of the situation at hand.

Although the evidence is mounting (O'Sullivan et al 1997, Hides et al 2001, Stuge et al 2004) and the principles behind the approach are sound, it should not be blindly prescribed for all individuals with LPD. Clinical reasoning must prevail. It is crucial that a therapist be able to identify the point in the rehabilitation process when motor control retraining is appropriate, and then to approach it in a way that addresses the individual needs of the patient. If this is not done both the patient and the therapist will become frustrated, and confidence in the approach, as well as the science upon which it is based, will be lost. For instance, the ability to accurately isolate and coordinate the deep muscle system cannot occur unless the neurophysiological environment is conducive. Ultimately, consideration must be given to the stage of healing of any damaged tissue, the presence of hypomobility secondary to joint or neuromeningeal restrictions, and the amount and cause of global muscle hypertonicity in the region before specific deficits of the deep muscle system can be effectively addressed. Individuals in the acute stages of healing, those with joint or neuromeningeal hypomobility, or hypertonicity of regional muscles secondary to these or other factors (cognitive, neurophysiological), are in most cases not appropriate for motor control retraining. Educational, manual or electrophysical techniques must first be used to address these issues. Once addressed, motor control retraining (augmented with USI) aimed at eliminating any residual hypertonicity, followed by facilitation of specific deep system muscles, and ultimately functional movement patterns will be of lasting value.

THE ROLE OF RTUS IN THE TREATMENT OF LUMBOPELVIC DYSFUNCTION

There is evidence from behavioural, functional imaging, electro-physiological as well as cellular and molecular studies suggesting that motor learning occurs in stages (Luft & Buitrago 2005). Furthermore, that progression through the stages is dependent upon the availability of different resources or types of information (Eversheim & Bock 2001). Several authors (Fitts 1964, Adams 1971, Shiffrin & Schneider 1977, Anderson 1982) have proposed models which are variable in number and characteristics of stages. Fitts (1964) described a three-stage model in which the first stage, referred to as the 'cognitive' or 'declarative' stage, is characterized by the individual striving to comprehend the rules, requirements and strategies involved in the task. The second stage, defined as the 'motor' or 'associative' stage, involves the gradual development of a fluent motor response with the help of sensory feedback (Eversheim & Bock 2001). The third and final stage is termed the 'autonomous' stage and is characterized by the task becoming automatic, rapid and capable of being integrated into larger motor sequences with greater immunity to disruption (Rosenbaum et al 2001).

Using a staged model as a framework to normalize motor control in the lumbopelvic region highlights that the needs of the cognitive and associative stages must be satisfied if progression onto the autonomous stage is to occur. As the real-time nature of USI allows the patient and therapist to view a muscle contraction (and its impact on surrounding structures) directly, it is a unique tool which can contribute novel and previously unavailable resources to fulfilment of these requirements. Consequently, RTUS can play two major roles in the treatment of motor control dysfunction in the lumbopelvic region. First during the cognitive stage, by providing play-by-play information which the therapist can use to educate a patient regarding their precise problem (what is actually happening within their bodies), as well as the specifics of the task at hand. Then secondly, during the associative stage as a form of biofeedback upon which a motor control performance can be modified, once an environment conducive for addressing it has been achieved.

Generally, restoration of motor control, or motor learning, within the lumbopelvic region will focus on either diminishing excessive or, facilitating and coordinating insufficient muscle activity during a particular task (resting posture, preferential activation, arm lift, leg lift, cough, sneeze, squat etc.). Whether an inhibitory or facilitatory strategy is chosen is dependent upon individual patient presentation. It is inappropriate to assume that the decision to inhibit or facilitate muscle activity can be made from an USI assessment alone. However, as a general rule, if an excessive response (see the end of Chapter 3) is identified, then inhibition of unwarranted muscle activity is likely appropriate, whereas identification of an insufficient response will likely indicate treatment aimed at facilitation or coordination of muscle activity. Clinically, it is common to find a combination of these factors at play; consequently, thorough consideration of all assessment findings in conjunction with vigilant definition of the impairment are required before an appropriate rehabilitation strategy can be devised (Lee 2004).

The use of RTUS for patient education (cognitive stage)

It is impossible to change a behaviour that we are not aware of or do not acknowledge, and it is difficult to acknowledge a behaviour that we cannot see, feel or, directly experience. If the behaviour is overt, such as performing a squatting motion, direct awareness is possible. We can reflect back on a performance, as well as receive sensory feedback during the task to cognitively analyse and modify the behaviour. However, this cognitive process is thwarted if the behaviour in question is ambiguous, such as unnecessary resting hyperactivity of the lateral abdominal wall muscles, an inability to preferentially activate the left side of the PFM, or the ability to sustain activity of the lumbar multifidus during a leg press exercise. As the concepts are foreign and unfamiliar there is likely to be a lack of awareness, and the individual will be unable to acknowledge and consequently successfully modify the behaviour. In the case of hypertonic lateral abdominal wall muscles the therapist may pass on that they have identified an inappropriate relaxation of certain muscles, explain what resting hypertonicity is, and perhaps even point out that the lack of trunk mobility and lateral costal expansion with respiration, as well as the trigger points in the patient's oblique abdominal muscles, are all indicators of this lack of relaxation. However, it is unlikely that a patient who feels that they are fully relaxed is going to truly experience the hypertonicity (the inappropriate behaviour that needs to be addressed) based entirely on the therapist's efforts, without first-hand awareness.

The merit of RTUS is that it allows a therapist to provide direct proof of the ambiguous behaviour to the patient, and perhaps more importantly, for the patient to experience it directly. For example, the patient can draw awareness to, and view the behaviour of the muscle in question during a motion that requires it to contract, and then with attempted relaxation. This process provides a level of awareness and understanding that is beyond compare and that has been found to be invaluable to the rehabilitation process. Consequently, once the assessment has been completed, the therapist should provide the patient with a clear and concise interpretation of the ultrasound image or images that most vividly demonstrate their dysfunction (e.g. image the lateral abdominal wall muscles during an ASLR and point out that they do not fully relax after the leg is returned to rest, or image the bladder and the impact or lack thereof with an attempted contraction of the PFM, etc.). This process should involve education on the anatomy, location and role of the muscles that are important for force closure of the region, as well as the specific dysfunction identified (insufficient vs. excessive response). As the conceptualization of the patient's dysfunction with the assistance of RTUS is a direct and interactive experience, it also encourages active participation and serves as a source of motivation.

The role of RTUS for feedback (cognitive and associative stages)

Progression through and the quality of the performance during each of the motor learning stages, as well as the degree of motor learning that ultimately occurs, will be influenced by the type and presentation of information about the performance, both during and after attempts made to achieve a specific goal (e.g. relaxing the left side of the PFM, or preferential activation of TrA). Feedback, biofeedback, knowledge of results and knowledge of performance are four types of information that are critical for modifying a motor response (Salmoni et al 1984).

Feedback refers to the information provided by the various sensory organs (eyes, ears, nose, mouth, proprioceptive organs, thermal receptors etc.) before, during and after a task, while biofeedback refers to signals that tell of what is happening within the body itself. Specific to restoration of motor control in the lumbopelvic region feedback can take the form of tactile information (from palpation of the muscles that should either be or not be involved in the task), visual information (from observation of the task) or kinaesthetic information (how did the task feel). However, when it comes to novel tasks such as relaxation of a muscle that is hypertonic, the successful preferential activation of a muscle that is deep and not directly accessible from the body surface, or optimizing a synergy of muscle contractions to achieve a particular task, traditional forms of feedback may not be sufficient and the unparalleled visual information (not to mention real-time biofeedback) available with RTUS can be a positive adjunct.

Knowledge of results (KR) refers to the information provided after the attempt of a motor performance that tells an individual of their success or failure in achieving their goal, and is viewed as the most important variable (except possibly practice) for learning. KR is information that is not naturally available from feedback alone, rather is a verbal statement about the outcome of an attempt (successful vs. unsuccessful) as opposed to its characteristics (the task was performed too quickly or with too great of an effort), which are termed knowledge of performance (KP) (Salmoni et al 1984). Both KR and KP are of great value to the motor learning process; however, their benefits can only be realized if they are available. There are various suggested methods of determining if there is a coordinated isometric co-contraction of the deep muscles, in conjunction with appropriate (dependent on the nature of the task) activation of the superficial muscles, which results in sufficient tension of the regional fascia, allowing for support of the pelvic viscera and skeletal system (Lee 2004). However, none provides the degree of detail or objectivity of information that is available with USI. Consequently, its incorporation exponentially enhances the quality of the information that is available to the patient, and diminishes the amount of time required to learn a task (Dietz et al 2001, Henry & Westervelt 2005).

Understanding how KR, KP and feedback improve motor learning provides a basis for recognizing the unique role that RTUS can play in this process, as well as for understanding the most advantageous way in which it should be incorporated. Various theories have been put forward with respect to how KR works; however, the three most relevant are that it plays a motivational or energizing role, that it serves to recalibrate an individual's internal scale of awareness, and that it acts as a form of guidance during the learning process. Salmoni et al (1984) points out that individuals who have access to KR are more interested in the task at hand, work harder at perfecting the task, and persist longer after KR is absent. KR may also serve as a mechanism by which the awareness of a region of the body can be recalibrated. Specifically, there is evidence to suggest that the internal scale of awareness of movement is often distorted with dysfunction (Moseley 2003), and that repeated exposure to KR during subsequent movements can serve as a basis upon which this distorted internal balance can been restored (Salmoni et al 1984). Finally, KR provides a strong guidance function for future performances through the identification of errors which become the basis upon which an individual can modify and improve the accuracy of their next attempt (Salmoni et al 1984). Although the literature suggests that several of these effects may only be temporary, they are consistent with clinical observations and likely begin to explain the potent affect that RTUS can have on motor learning.

The value of feedback and KR on motor learning can be enhanced if care is given to their presentation. Specifically, motor learning has been shown to be inferior in situations in which KR and feedback are given on every trial of a task, as opposed to situations in which trials that do not provide this information are interspersed (Salmoni et al 1984). These findings suggest that due to its guiding role, patients may concentrate or rely too heavily on KR and consequently degrade learning. Therefore, clinical situations that intersperse RTUS feedback and KR are more likely to enhance motor learning than situations that do not. Furthermore, motor learning has been shown to be superior in situations in which intruding thought processes and distractions are minimized, where there is adequate time between trials to analyse the feedback from the previous attempt, when KR and feedback are precise and explicit, as well as when there has been greater variability in practice conditions (Salmoni et al 1984).

Clinically, whether RTUS is being used in an attempt to normalize muscle hypertonicity, or to facilitate muscle activity, the concepts surrounding the stages of motor learning, as well as the role and principles of optimal presentation of KR and feedback should be kept in mind. As suggested above, the incorrect activation strategies identified in Chapter 3 considered in conjunction with findings from the rest of the assessment process serve to direct the focus of treatment. If the findings indicate an excessive motor control response, then the focus of treatment will likely be aimed at reducing hypertonicity, while if they point to an insufficient response, then the aim will be to facilitate muscle activity or synergy.

The use of RTUS to reduce hypertonicity

The presence of unnecessary muscle activity for a given loading situation is a defining characteristic of an excessive motor control strategy. This will be demonstrated on USI as either an inability to fully relax a muscle(s) in a resting situation (**Figs 3.1b, 3.15a, 3.16b, 5.2a**), resting respiratory modulation of the abdominal wall (**Fig. 3.2a, b**), an inability to demonstrate preferential activation of a specific muscle (**Figs 3.7a, 3.13b, 3.22a, b**), excessive activation during, or an inability to fully relax a muscle(s) at the completion of a task.

The first step in normalizing excessive muscle activity is to understand why it exists. Generally, hypertonicity is in response to a perceived threat; however, if left unchallenged it can persist once the threat has diminished, and become maladaptive and a potential source of symptoms (O'Sullivan 2005). Consequently, every attempt must be made to identify and address any and all potential threats, regardless of whether they are biomechanical (hypomobility due to articular or neuromeningeal restriction), patho-anatomical (structural disruptions such as spondylolithesis and loss of fascial integrity), cognitive (fear avoidance, lack of strategies for coping with pain) or neurophysiological (chemical inflammation, central or peripheral sensitization of the sensory system, as well as altered regulation of pH resulting from hypocapnia) in nature, as until this is done, little lasting change of an excessive motor control strategy will be seen. Attempting to minimize muscle hypertonicity through the use of RTUS (as a form of feedback and KR) alone is unlikely to address the underlying driving forces. Consequently, the most appropriate form of treatment may include anti–inflammatory medication, joint mobilization or manipulation, neuromeningeal mobilization, trigger point release and restoration of respiratory mechanics, as well as education on habitual movement patterns or postures, neutral spine, topics surrounding pain beliefs, basis for a fear of motion and neurophysiology prior to, or in conjunction with, RTUS. The specific technique, or combination of techniques chosen, will depend entirely on the specific presentation of the patient (Butler 2000, Chaitow et al 2002, Lee 2004).

If all sources of inflammation, as well as joint and neuromeningeal restriction, have been eliminated, a persisting inability to fully relax a muscle in a resting state is an indicator for a treatment approach that incorporates respiration and relaxation strategies. However, associated with these tactics, an effort should be made to identify any missing or inappropriate cognitive or neurophysiological beliefs, as well as to incorporate techniques (dry needling, tripper point pressure release) aimed at reducing trigger points in the hypertonic muscles (Butler & Moseley 2003, Lee 2004, Thorn 2004). If the muscles of the region can be relaxed, but there is a persisting inability to separate the deep and superficial muscles with preferential activation, it is likely that an approach which incorporates either an indirect facilitatory technique (see below under the role of RTUS in the facilitation of muscle activity) and/or more explicit definition of the task at hand is indicated. In such cases it is useful to encourage the patient to provide an explanation of their understanding of the task and then use the details to guide what information needs to be provided or clarified. Furthermore, if preferential activation can be consistently achieved, yet an excessive timing issue (either premature, disproportionate or excessive activation during, and/or an inability to fully relax a muscle at the completion of, a task) persists, it is likely that a treatment approach focused on cognitively breaking down and increasing the awareness of the task and the muscle's response during the task is required.

RTUS can serve as an adjunct in all of the above scenarios by displaying the subtleties of muscle behaviour so that they can be discussed and modified. Although the methodology employed can be as varied as the unique characteristics of a patient (e.g. symmetrical or asymmetrical hypertonicity of the pelvic floor, vs.

abdominal obliques, vs. thoracolumbar erector spinae), or the creativity of a therapist, there are general concepts that can serve as guidelines. An example of a method that utilizes RTUS to assist in diminishing an excessive motor control strategy of the lateral abdominal wall muscles will be used to demonstrate these underlying principles.

The use of RTUS to reduce hypertonicity of the lateral abdominal wall muscles

The first step in minimizing hypertonicity is to ensure that the patient is at ease and that all potential threats (physical, cognitive and emotional) have been addressed. This involves consideration of the general environment (noise level, temperature and exposure) and the therapist's approach (calm, soft spoken, compassionate and relaxed), as well as the patient's receptivity. The patient should be placed in a position that is comfortable, produces minimal symptoms or undue load on any specific structure, and requires little to no effort to maintain. If appropriate, attention should be given to the influence of gravity on the body, as well as the possibility for visual (view of the ultrasound screen) and tactile (hand on their belly) access to the hypertonic region (stomach and lateral costal region). In the case of a hypertonic abdominal wall, a side-lying posture that incorporates adequate support of the neck and thoracolumbar junction is often effective. However, it is important to keep in mind that every patient presentation and clinical situation is unique, and the ideal position will change accordingly.

Often individuals that demonstrate a high degree of hypertonicity are unable to maintain any one position for a sustained period of time. Consequently, changes of position or movement breaks may need to be interspersed within the feedback session. Once the individual has indicated that they are comfortable in the side-lying position, their bottom arm should be wrapped around their trunk so that their hand can encompass the uppermost lateral costal region. The top hand is then free to encompass the lower abdominal region (**Fig. 5.1a**). The nature of this set-up maximizes the learning environment by providing tactile information from both the lateral costal region and lower abdomen, as well as the potential for visual feedback (ultrasound screen), KR and KP when USI is added to the set-up (**Fig. 5.1b**).

Once an appropriate patient position has been achieved, several strategies can be employed to address lateral abdominal wall hypertonicity. However, as respiration is a physiological priority the initial focus should centre on decreasing the expiratory effort coming from the abdominal wall muscles. This involves ensuring that any factors resulting in decreased passive recoil of the thorax or contributing to exaggerated respiration have been addressed,

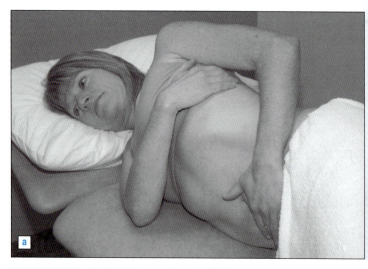

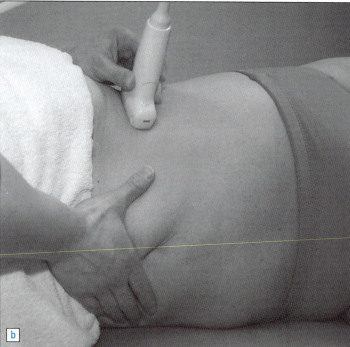

Figure 5.1 Reducing hypertonicity of the lateral abdominal wall. **a.** A side-lie position that optimizes tactile (thorax and abdominal wall) and visual feedback (when USI is added to the set-up). **b.** Kinaesthetic facilitation of abdominal wall relaxation in association with RTUS feedback. The patient is encouraged to relax their abdominal wall into the therapist's hand while attending to the changes to the muscle layers on the ultrasound screen.

followed by bringing attention to the pattern (location of expansion, rate and frequency, ratio of inspiration to expiration as well as the status of an expiratory pause) of respiration that the patient is using. If the contributory factors have been addressed, then the patient should be encouraged to bring awareness to where they are breathing in their body, by attending to the tactile information from their hands, as well as their thorax against the bed. If there is obvious resting respiratory modulation visible on the ultrasound screen it should be pointed out to the patient. The patient can then experiment between lateral costal vs. abdominal expansion during inspiration and observe the impact that these different strategies have on the respiratory modulation. Generally, abdominal expansion will result in greater respiratory modulation (as the abdominal contents are pushed out into the lateral abdominal wall muscles), while lateral costal expansion followed by a passive expiration will result in less. The patient should focus on attaining a resting respiratory pattern that ensures some lateral costal expansion during inspiration, a slow (equal in length to inspiration) relaxed expiration resulting from passive recoil of the rib cage (as opposed to abdominal muscle activity), followed by a brief expiratory pause, while attending to the visual information from the ultrasound screen and the tactile information from their hands and thorax, as well as the instruction and feedback coming from the therapist. As the patient gains control over their respiratory pattern using the feedback from the RTUS, it should be intermittently removed, and the relaxation internalized. Moreover, when appropriate the resting respiratory pattern should be practised in a variety of other positions (e.g. supine lie, prone lie, reclined and unsupported sitting). If improving the balance between lateral costal and abdominal expansion, as well as eliminating any forced expiration fails to impact the resting respiratory modulation, then it is possible that the cause is related to chemical drive and likely will require further investigation (e.g. capnography) (Chaitow et al 2002, Whittaker 2005).

Once control over the resting respiratory pattern has been accomplished, focus should switch to maintaining the pattern while allowing the abdominal muscles to relax and the belly hang out. The therapist can place emphasis on both an image and a sensation of the abdominal contents falling onto the innermost surface of TrA, as well as the consequential change in the ultrasound image (a decrease in width and increase in length of the lateral abdominal wall muscle layers) which corresponds to relaxation (**Fig. 5.2a, b**). The letting go of the abdominal wall muscles can be further facilitated by the therapist gently encompassing the patient's lower abdominal contents, supporting them back into the abdomen, and then encouraging relaxation with the assistance of gravity when the support of the hand is removed and the abdominal contents fall back out (**Fig. 5.1b**). As the patient becomes successful in relaxing

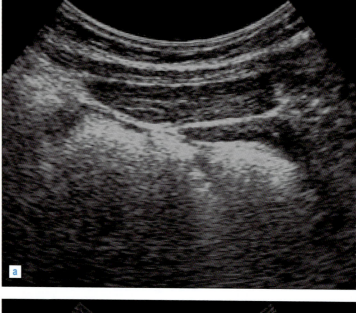

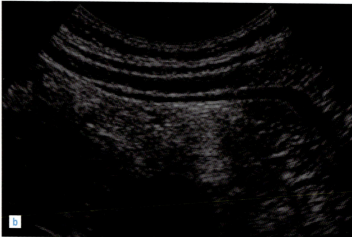

Figure 5.2 Reducing hypertonicity of the lateral abdominal wall. **a.** An ultrasound image of resting hypertonicity of the right lateral abdominal wall. **b.** An ultrasound image of the same abdominal wall post-treatment. As the patient learns to relax their abdominal wall they will see a corresponding increase in length and decrease in width of the muscle layers on the ultrasound screen.

the lateral abdominal wall muscles using the feedback from the RTUS, it should be intermittently removed, and the relaxation internalized. Moreover, when appropriate the ability to relax the lateral abdominal wall while preserving an appropriate resting respiratory pattern should be practised in a variety of positions (e.g. supine lie, prone lie, reclined sitting, and unsupported sitting).

Once an individual can consistently demonstrate relaxation of the lateral abdominal wall muscles without visual (RTUS) or tactile feedback in a variety of positions, they are ready to address any deficits in the anterior component of the deep muscle system.

The use of RTUS to facilitate muscle activity

The absence of adequate muscle activity for a given loading situation is a defining characteristic of an insufficient motor control strategy. This will manifest itself on USI as either a hypotonic muscle contraction (either symmetrically or asymmetrically), an incompetent muscle contraction (due either to length tension issues of the muscle itself, or as a result of insufficient muscle bulk within a fascial compartment) (**Fig. 3.6b**), incompetent fascia (**Fig. 3.10b**), or as a timing deficiency in which there is either delayed or inconsistent (premature loss) activation of a muscle(s) during a task (**Fig. 3.4c**). Once any hypertonicity in the region has been addressed, the first step in normalizing an insufficient motor control strategy is to understand the specific deficiency of the patient in question. However, as the clinical presentation may change once the unwarranted activity is addressed, and as the underlying neurophysiological dysfunction may involve multiple deep, or for that matter superficial, system muscles, ongoing assessment is critical.

If the insufficiency is due to activation, bulk or timing deficiencies of a muscle, or group of muscles, the patient is likely to benefit from treatment aimed at activating and then coordinating the function of the deficient muscle(s) with other muscles in the region. If the insufficiency is primarily due to fascial concerns (lengthened or disrupted) the treatment approach is similar; however, the prognosis is slower, and in extreme situations may require referral to surgical consultation. The facilitation of a muscle, or group of muscles, can be greatly enhanced with RTUS and often can be accomplished in a rudimentary fashion within a few minutes. Although the methodology employed can be as varied as the specific needs of a patient (e.g. ineffective activation of the PFM, or ineffective activation of the right TrA associated with insufficiency of the left dMF) or the creativity of a therapist, there are general concepts that can serve as guidelines. An example of a method that utilizes RTUS to assist in facilitating activation of TrA will be used to demonstrate these underlying principles.

The use of RTUS for the activation and coordination of TrA

The first step in facilitating activation of a muscle is to ensure that the patient is at ease, and that all potential distractions (physical, cognitive and emotional) have been addressed. This involves consideration of the general environment (noise level, temperature, exposure), the therapist's approach (calm, soft spoken, relaxed) and patient's receptivity. The patient should be placed in a position that is comfortable, produces minimal symptoms or undue load on any specific structure, and requires little to no effort to maintain. If appropriate, attention should be given to the influence of gravity on the body, as well as the possibility for visual (view of the ultrasound screen) and tactile (hand on their belly) access to the region of interest (stomach and lateral costal region). In the case of facilitating activation of the TrA, a side-lying posture that incorporates adequate support of the neck and thoracolumbar junction has been found to be advantageous. However, it is important to keep in mind that every patient presentation and clinical situation is unique, and the ideal position will change accordingly.

Once the individual has indicated that they are comfortable in the side-lying position their bottom arm should be wrapped around their trunk so that their hand can encompass the uppermost lateral costal region. The top hand is then free to encompass the lower abdominal region (**Fig. 5.1a**). The nature of this set-up maximizes the learning environment by providing tactile information from both the lateral costal region and lower abdomen, as well as the potential for visual feedback (ultrasound screen), KR and KP when RTUS is added to the set-up (**Fig. 5.3a**).

Prior to attempting a contraction an explicit definition of the task at hand should be provided to the patient. This may involve a review of the anatomy of the region and what happens when the muscle(s) contracts (no spinal motion, abdominal contents retracting), as well as the desired speed and effort of the contraction. It is useful to encourage the patient to provide an explanation of their understanding of the task and use this to guide further clarification or provision of information. Once the patient has a clear understanding of the task at hand, several strategies can be employed to facilitate an isolated contraction of TrA. Either a direct (involving

---

Figure 5.3 Activation and coordination of TrA. **a.** A side-lying position that optimizes tactile (thorax and abdominal wall) and visual feedback (RTUS). In this scenario the therapist is providing kinaesthetic facilitation combined with RTUS feedback aimed at encouraging preferential activation of TrA through gently drawing in the lower abdominal wall. **b.** Preferential activation followed by coordinated co-contraction of the deep muscle system during a single leg drop in a supine position. In this scenario the patient first practises preferential activation of TrA followed by tonic activation coordinated with the rest of the deep muscle system during a single leg drop. Note that the patient is gathering tactile information with both their left (IO/TrA) and right (thorax expansion with inspiration) hands, while attending to the visual feedback being provided by RTUS.

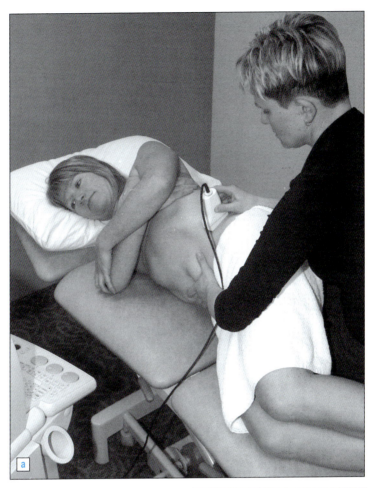

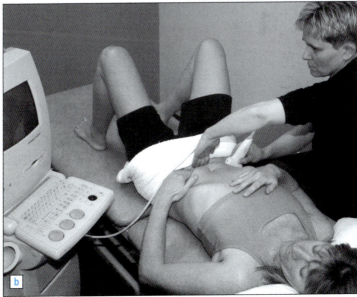

the abdominal wall) or an indirect approach (involving another deep system muscle or an image) may prove useful.

A direct approach involves drawing attention to inward motion of the lower abdominal wall independent of any posterior pelvic tilting, thoracolumbar flexion or breath holding. The therapist can facilitate this by gently encompassing the lower abdominal region (below the umbilicus) of the patient, and physically encouraging the abdominal contents back into the abdomen (**Fig. 5.3a**). This passive motion is followed by active assisted and eventually active attempts by the patient to mimic this action. During the passive component of this strategy the patient is encouraged to attend to their lower abdomen as the therapist manipulates the region (e.g. the direction in which the lower abdominal region is moving, the speed at which it is moving and the excursion of the motion). The therapist takes care to produce slow, inward (not up or downward) motion of the lower abdominal region (below the umbilicus) with relatively little excursion. After a couple of passive repetitions the patient is encouraged to gently assist with the drawing in motion. At this point the patient brings their attention to the ultrasound screen and the therapist points out successes (a slow and controlled increase in the depth, decrease in the length, and lateral corseting of TrA while it slides under a resting IO) (**Fig. 3.5a, b**) and failures (KR), as well as information that can be used to guide and modify future attempts (KP) (**Fig. 5.3a, b**). As the patient begins to grasp the motor control skill they progress to submaximal tonic holding, followed by controlled relaxation with use of the RTUS as feedback. Once the patient can do this and coordinate the holding phase with resting respiration then the feedback should be intermittently removed and control over the task internalized.

An indirect approach would involve identifying if an isolated contraction of one of the other deep system muscles, such as the PFM (Sapsford et al 2001), or a specific image ('imagine there is a wire connecting your hip bones together anteriorly from the left to right side; think about generating a force which would draw these two bones together') (Lee 2004) result in a concurrent co-contraction of TrA. If this is the case, then either the PFM or imagery cue can be used to indirectly facilitate the TrA through a similar progression. Clinically, the indirect approach is useful as a method to draw attention away from the action of the abdominal wall muscles if there is a tendency for hyperactivity in the region (e.g. oblique abdominals). A similar approach would be to use an abdominal strategy to facilitate the dMF if there is a tendency for hypertonicity of the thoracolumbar extensors with a lumbar cue. While an indirect approach is a very useful strategy during the initial stages of 'waking up a muscle', it is important to note that in the case of the TrA and PFM, there has been some suggestion that independent control is eventually preferable. Although this topic is somewhat controversial, there appears to be substantial clinical support for the concept that during bowel evacuation or delivery it is advantageous if the PFM can fully relax while the TrA can be used to increase intra-abdominal pressure (de Gasquet & Valancogne 2001).

It is important to understand that there are a variety of kinaesthetic or verbal cues, as well as images, that can be used to elicit preferential activation of the deep muscle system (see Chapter 3). Although a cue or image may be successful with some patients, the assumption that they will work for all is faulty and commonly a therapist will develop a repertoire of several options that they find have the most clinical utility. If improving the understanding of the task, optimizing feedback and attempting both direct and indirect cues fails to improve the ability of the individual to preferentially activate a muscle, then it is likely that there has been a breakdown in communication between the therapist and patient, or that the neurophysiological environment is not conducive and further investigation is required.

If, however, the patient can demonstrate preferential activation of the muscle of interest (TrA), regardless of whether a direct or indirect cue is used, the primary goal is to hold the contraction for a short period of time (10-20s), in a submaximal fashion, while preserving resting respiration. As the patient becomes successful at this with the assistance of verbal, tactile and visual feedback (RTUS), then the feedback should be intermittently removed, and the contraction internalized. At this point in the progression it is important that the patient begin to coordinate the isolated muscle effort with the rest of the deep system muscles. If an insufficiency of another of the deep system muscles had previously been detected, it is at this point that both are reintegrated. Once a coordinated contraction of the deep muscle system (including respiration) independent of feedback, in the initial posture, has been attained, the patient can progress to performing the co-contraction in a variety of other positions (supine lie, prone lie, reclined sitting, unsupported sitting and standing) (**Fig. 5.3b**). If the patient demonstrates a tendency to bring in excessive (actual amount or at inappropriate times) superficial muscle activity (some may be expected with unsupported and standing) with increased effort or enthusiasm, then the impact of this on the ultrasound image should be pointed out. The goal in doing so is to improve the patient's awareness of exactly what this inappropriate effort feels like, and when it is occurring so that it can be modified.

Once a coordinated contraction of the deep muscle system, independent of feedback, can be demonstrated in a variety of positions, the patient is ready to begin integrating the deep and superficial muscle systems during tasks that perturb the region (limb motion) (**Fig. 5.3b**) and are more functional in nature (such as squatting, lunging etc.) (**Fig. 5.4a, b**). This reintegration should involve an increasingly challenging progression of tasks which ultimately end with functional movement experiences with specific importance to the patient (Richardson et al 2004, Lee 2004). If the individual reverts to either an insufficient (hypoactivity, delayed, inconsistent or premature loss) or excessive (hyperactive, premature, inability to fully relax) response (identified with RTUS) during a task at any point in the progression the motion should be cognitively broken down and awareness brought to the point in the sequence where motor control is lost so that the response can be modified. Again, once the individual can perform the functional movements with the assistance of RTUS, then the feedback should be intermittently removed and control over the task internalized (**Fig. 5.4b**).

As mentioned above, the specific techniques that can be employed to either reduce hypertonicity and unwarranted muscle activity (excessive motor control response), or to facilitate and coordinate a specific muscle or group of muscles (insufficient motor control response) can be as varied as the specific needs of the patient and creativity of the therapist. The general concepts that underlie the process have been demonstrated with respect to the abdominal wall. However, they can easily be extrapolated to the paraspinal and

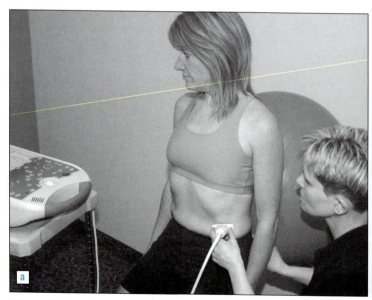

Figure 5.4 Functional progression of TrA activation. **a.** Initially the patient performs a supported wall squat while integrating visual feedback from RTUS to ensure that she is maintaining tonic activation of TrA (in association with a coordinated co-contraction of the rest of the deep muscle system) throughout.

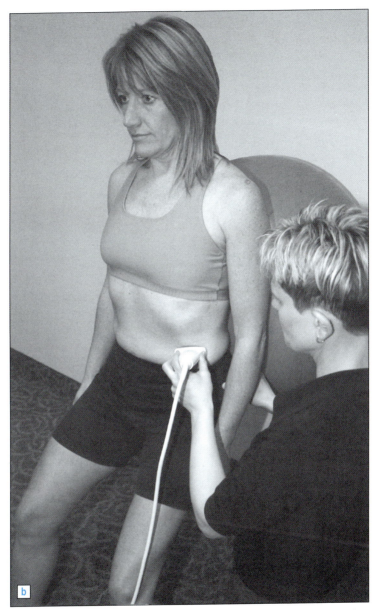

Figure 5.4, Cont'd b. Once the patient can consistently maintain tonic activation of their TrA with the aid of visual feedback it is intermittently removed (they turn their head away or close their eyes) and the skill is internalized.

pelvic floor regions, as well as more complicated clinical presentations (e.g. one in which there is a deficiency in several of the local system muscles).

CONCLUSION

In conclusion, this chapter is not intended as a comprehensive guide for the treatment of lumbopelvic dysfunction, rather as a summary of the fundamental concepts underlying the clinical integration of RTUS in the treatment of motor control dysfunction in the lumbopelvic region. In particular, the goal was to clarify under what conditions and by what means the use of RTUS is appropriate. Finally, it is important for those considering, and who are employing RTUS for treatment, to understand that it is not intended as a stand-alone intervention, rather as one (although be it extremely valuable) tool in a multi-modal management approach (see Appendix C – case presentation).

References

Abe T, Kusuhara N, Yoshimura N et al 1996 Differential respiratory activity of four abdominal muscles in humans. Journal of Applied Physiology 80(4):1379-1389

Adams J A 1971 A closed loop theory of motor learning. Journal of Motor Behavior 3:111-149

Ainscough-Potts A M, Morrissey M C, Critchley D 2006 The response of the transverse abdominis and internal oblique muscles to different postures. Manual Therapy 11(1):54-60

AIUM 2000 American institute of ultrasound in medicine official statements and reports. Online. Available: http://www.aium.org

Amonoo-Kuofi H S 1983 The density of muscle spindles in the medial, intermediate and lateral columns of human intrinsic postvertebral muscles. Journal of Anatomy 136:509-519

Andary M T, Hallgren R C, Greenman P F et al 1998 Neurogenic atrophy of suboccipital muscle after a cervical injury: a case study. American Journal of Physical Medicine and Rehabilitation 77:545-549

Anderson J R 1982 Acquisition of cognitive skill. Psychological Review 89:369-406

Aston-Miller J A, Howard D, DeLancey J O L 2001 The functional anatomy of the female pelvic floor and stress continence control system. Scandinavian Journal of Urology and Nephrology Supplementum 207:1-7

Barbic M, Kralj B, Cor A 2003 Compliance of the bladder neck supporting structures: Importance of activity pattern of levator ani muscle and content of elastic fibers of endopelvic fascia. Neurourology and Urodynamics 22:269-273

Beer-Gabel M, Teshler M, Barzilai N et al 2002 Dynamic transperineal ultrasound in the diagnosis of pelvic floor disorders: pilot study. Diseases of the Colon and Rectum 45:239-248

Bergmark A 1989 Stability of the lumbar spine. A study in mechanical engineering. Acta Orthopaedica Scandinavian Supplementum 230(60): 20-24

Bernstein I, Juul N, Gronvall S et al 1991 Pelvic floor muscle thickness measured by perineal ultrasonography. Scandinavian Journal of Urology and Nephrology Supplementum 137:131-133

Blaney F, English C S, Sawyer T 1999 Sonographic measurement of diaphragmatic displacement during tidal breathing maneuvers – A reliability study. Australian Journal of Physiotherapy 45:41-43

Bø K, Stein R 1994 Needle EMG registration of striated urethral wall and pelvic floor muscle activity patterns during cough, valsalva, abdominal, hip adductor, and gluteal muscles contractions in nulliparous healthy females. Neurourology and Urodynamics 13:35-41

Bø K, Lilleas F, Talseth T et al 2001 Dynamic MRI of the pelvic floor muscles in an upright sitting position. Neurourology and Urodynamics 20:167-174

Bø K, Sherburn M, Allen T 2003 Transabdominal ultrasound measurement of pelvic floor muscle activity when activated directly or via a transversus abdominis muscle contraction. Neurourology and Urodynamics 22:582-588

Bunce S M, Moore A P, Hough A D 2002 M-mode ultrasound: a reliable measure of transversus abdominis thickness? Clinical Biomechanics 17:315-317

Bunce S M, Hough A D, Moore A P 2004 Measurement of abdominal muscle thickness using M-mode ultrasound imaging during functional activities. Manual Therapy 9:41-44

Butler D S 2000 The sensitive nervous system. Noigroup Publications, Adelaide

Butler D S, Moseley L G 2003 Explain pain. Noigroup Publications, Adelaide

Campbell S E, Alder R, Sofka C M 2005 Ultrasound of muscle abnormalities. Ultrasound Quarterly 21(2):87-94

Chaitow L, Bradley D, Gilbert C 2002 Multidisciplinary approaches to breathing pattern disorders. Churchill Livingstone, Edinburgh

Cholewicki J C, Silfies S P, Shah R A et al 2005 Delayed trunk muscle reflex responses increase the risk of low back injuries. Spine 30(23):2614-2620

Christensen L L, Djurhuus J C, Constantinou C E 1995 Imaging of pelvic floor contractions using MRI. Neurourology and Urodynamics 14(3): 209-216

Coldron Y, Stokes M, Cook K 2003 Lumbar multifidus muscles size does not differ whether ultrasound imaging is performed in prone or side lying. Manual Therapy 8(3):161-165

Constantinou C E, Govan D E 1982 Spatial distribution and timing of transmitted and reflexly generated urethral pressures in healthy women. Journal of Urology 127:964-969

Cowan S M, Schache A G, Brukner P et al 2004 Delayed onset of transversus abdominis in long-standing groin pain. Medicine & Science in Sports & Exercise Dec:2040-2045

Crichley D J, Coutts F J 2002 Abdominal muscle function in chronic low back pain patients, measurement with real-time ultrasound scanning. Physiotherapy June 88(6):322-332

Deindl F M, Vodusek D B, Hesse U et al 1994 Pelvic floor activity pattern: comparison of nulliparous continent and parous urinary stress incontinent women. A kinesiological EMG study. British Journal of Urology 73:413-417

de Gasquet B, Valancogne G 2001 La poussée défécatoire. In: Jauze R (eds) Constipations solutions. Paris, France, p 117-121

Delitto A 2005 Research in low back pain time to stop seeking the elusive "magic bullet." Physical Therapy 85(3):206-208

DeTroyer A, Estenne M, Ninane V et al 1990 Transversus abdominis muscle function in humans. Journal of Applied Physiology 68(3): 1010-1016

Dietz H P, Wilson P D 1999 The influence of bladder volume on the position and mobility of the urethrovesical junction. International Urogynecology Journal 10:3-6

Dietz H P, Clarke B 2001 The influence of posture on perineal ultrasound imaging parameters. International Urogynecology Journal 12:104-106

Dietz H P, Wilson P D, Clarke B 2001 The use of perineal ultrasound to quantify levator activity and teach pelvic floor muscle exercises. International Urogynecology Journal 12:166-169

Dietz H P, Jarvis S K, Vancaillie T G 2002 The assessment of levator muscle strength: a validation of three ultrasound techniques. International Urogynecology Journal 13:156-159

Dietz H P, Pang S, Korda A et al 2005 Paravaginal defects: a comparison of clinical examination and 2D/3D ultrasound imaging. Australian and New Zealand Journal of Obstetrics and Gynaecology 45:187-190

Elliott J M, Zylstra E D, Centeno C J 2004 Case Report: The presence and utilization of psoas musculature despite congenital absence of the right hip. Manual Therapy 9:109-113

Eversheim U, Bock O 2001 Evidence for processing stages in skill acquisition: a dual task study. Learning & Memory 8:183-189

Falla D, Bilenkij G, Jull G 2004a Patients with chronic neck pain demonstrate altered patterns of muscle activation during performance of a functional upper limb task. Spine 29(13):1436-1440

Falla D, Jull G, Hodges P W 2004b Feedforward activity of the cervical flexor muscles during voluntary arm movements is delayed in chronic neck pain. Experimental Brain Research 157:43-48

Ferreira P H, Ferreira M L, Hodges P W 2004 Changes in recruitment of the abdominal muscles in people with low back pain, ultrasound measurement of muscle activity. Spine 29(22):2560-2566

Fielding J R, Griffiths D J, Versi E et al 1998 MR imaging of pelvic floor continence mechanisms in the supine and sitting positions. American Journal of Roentgenology 171(6):1607-1610

Fitts P M 1964 Perceptual-motor skill learning. In: Melton A W (ed) Categories of human learning. Academic Press, New York, p 243-285

FitzGerald M P, Kotarinos R 2003a Rehabilitation of the short pelvic floor. I. Background and patient evaluation. International Urogynecology Journal 14:261-268

FitzGerald M P, Kotarinos R 2003b Rehabilitation of the short pelvic floor. II. Treatment of the patient with the short pelvic floor. International Urogynecology Journal 14:269-275

Gardner W N 1996 The pathophysiology of hyperventilation disorders. Chest 109:516-534

Gibbons S G T 2001 Biomechanics and stability mechanisms of psoas major. In: Proceedings of the 4th interdisciplinary world congress on low back and pelvic pain, Montreal, Canada, p 246

Gibbons S G T 2004 Functional anatomy of gluteus maximus: Deep sacral gluteus maximus – A new muscle? In: Proceedings of the 5th interdisciplinary world congress on low back and pelvic pain, Melbourne, Australia, p 54

Goldman J M, Lehr R P, Millar A B et al 1987 An electromyographic study of the abdominal muscles during postural and respiratory maneuvers. Journal of Neurourology, Neurosurgery and Psychiatry 50:866-869

Haberkorn U, Layer G, Ruday V et al 1993 Ultrasound image properties influenced by abdominal wall thickness and composition. Journal of Clinical Ultrasound 21:423-429

Hay-Smith E, Bø K, Berghmans L et al 2001 Pelvic floor muscle training for urinary incontinence in women (Cochrane review) 3. Oxford: The Cochrane Library

Hedrick W R 1995 Ultrasound physics and instrumentation, 3rd edn. Mosby, St. Louis

Hemborg B, Moritz U, Lowing H 1985 Intra-abdominal pressure and trunk muscle activity during lifting: IV. The causal factors of the intra-abdominal pressure rise. Scandinavian Journal of Rehabilitation Medicine 17(1):25-38

Henry S M, Westervelt K C 2005 The use of real-time ultrasound feedback in teaching abdominal hollowing exercises to healthy subjects. Journal of Orthopaedic & Sports Physical Therapy 36(6):338-345

Hides J, Cooper D H, Stokes M J 1992 Diagnostic ultrasound imaging for measurement of the lumbar multifidus muscle in normal young adults. Physiotherapy Theory and Practice 8:19-26

Hides J A, Stokes M J, Saide M et al 1994 Evidence of lumbar multifidus muscles wasting ipsilateral to symptoms in patients with acute/sub acute low back pain. Spine 19(2):165-177

Hides J, Richardson C A, Jull G A 1995a Magnetic resonance imaging and ultrasonography of the lumbar multifidus muscle; comparison of two different modalities. Spine 20(1):54-58

Hides J, Richardson C A, Jull G A et al 1995b Ultrasound imaging in rehabilitation. Australian Journal of Physiotherapy 41(3):187-193

Hides J A, Jull G A, Richardson C A 2001 Long term effects of specific stabilizing exercises for first episode low back pain. Spine 26(11): E243-E248

Hides J A, Wilson S, Stanton W et al 2006 An MRI investigation into the function of the transversus abdominis muscle during 'drawing in' of the abdominal wall. Spine 31(6):E175-E178

Hodges P W, Richardson C A 1996 Inefficient muscular stabilization of the lumbar spine associated with low back pain. A motor control evaluation of transversus abdominis. Spine 21(22):2640-2650

Hodges P W, Richardson C A, Jull G A 1996 Evaluation of the relationship between laboratory and clinical tests of transversus abdominis function. Physiotherapy Research International 1:30-40

Hodges P W, Richardson C A 1997 Feed forward contraction of transversus abdominis is not influenced by the direction of arm movement. Experimental Brain Research 114:362-370

Hodges P W, Butler J E, McKenzie D K et al 1997 Contraction of the human diaphragm during rapid postural adjustments. Journal of Physiology 505(2):539-548

Hodges P W, Gandevia S C 2000a Changes in intra-abdominal pressure during postural and respiratory activation of the human diaphragm. Journal of Applied Physiology 89:967-976

Hodges P W, Gandevia S C 2000b Activation of the human diaphragm during a repetitive postural task. Journal of Physiology 522(1):165-175

Hodges P W 2001 Changes in motor planning of feedforward postural responses of the trunk muscles in low back pain. Experimental Brain Research 141(2):261-266

Hodges P W, Heijnen I, Gandevia S C 2001 Postural activity of the diaphragm is reduced in humans when respiratory demand increases. Journal of Physiology 15;537(Pt 3):999-1008

Hodges P W, Sapsford R, Pengel L 2002 Feedforward activity of the pelvic floor muscles precedes rapid upper limb movements. Australian Physiotherapy Association Conference, Sydney, abstract 21

Hodges P W 2003 Core stability exercise in chronic low back pain. Orthopedic Clinics of North America 34:245-254

Hodges P W, Moseley L G 2003 Pain and motor control of the lumbopelvic region: effect and possible mechanisms. Journal of Electromyography and Kinesiology 13:361-370

Hodges P W, Pengel L H M, Herbert R D et al 2003a Measurement of muscle contraction with ultrasound imaging. Muscle and Nerve 27:682-692

Hodges P W, Kaigle Holm A, Holm S, Ekstrom L, Cresswell A G, Hansson T, Thorstensson A 2003b Intervertebral stiffness of the spine is increased by evoked contraction of transversus abdominis and the diaphragm: in vivo porcine studies. Spine Dec 1;28(23):2594-2601

Hodges P W 2005a Ultrasound imaging in rehabilitation: just a fad? Journal of Orthopaedic & Sports Physical Therapy 35(6):333-337

Hodges P W 2005b Why do exercise intervention work for low back pain. 2nd International Conference on Movement Dysfunction, Pain and Performance: Evidence and Effect, Edinburgh, UK

Hodges P W, Eriksson A E M, Shirley D et al 2005 Intra-abdominal pressure increases stiffness of the lumbar spine. Journal of Biomechanics 38:1873-1880

Hodgson T J, Collins M C 1991 Anterior abdominal wall hernias: diagnosis by ultrasound and tangential radiographs. Clinical Radiology 44:185-188

Houston J G, Angus R M, Cowan M D et al 1994 Ultrasound assessment of normal hemidiaphragmatic movement: relation to inspiratory volume. Thorax 49:500-503

Howard D, Miller J M, DeLancey J O L et al 2000 Differential effects of cough, valsalva, and continence status on vesicle neck movement. Obstetrics and Gynecology 95(4):535

Hungerford B, Gilleard W, Hodges P W 2003 Evidence of altered lumbopelvic muscle recruitment in the presence of sacroiliac joint pain. Spine 28(14):1593-1600

Hungerford B, Gilleard W, Lee D 2004 Altered patterns of pelvic bone motion determined in subjects with posterior pelvic pain using skin markers. Clinical Biomechanics 19:456-464

Jull G A, Richardson C A 2000 Motor control problems in patients with spinal pain: A new direction for therapeutic exercises. Journal of Manipulative and Physiological Therapeutics 23(2):115-117

Kader D F, Wardlaw D, Smith F W 2000 Correlation between the MRI changes in the lumbar multifidus muscles and leg pain. Clinical Radiology 55(2):145-149

Kermode F 2004 Benefits of utilizing real-time ultrasound imaging in the rehabilitation of the lumbar spine stabilizing muscles following low back injury in the elite athlete – a single case study. Physical Therapy in Sport 5:13-16

Kidd A W, Magee S, Richardson C A 2002 Reliability of real-time ultrasound for the assessment of transversus abdominis function. Journal of Gravitational Physiology 9(1):131-132

Kremkau F W 2002 Diagnostic ultrasound: Principles and instruments, 6th edn. Saunders, Philadelphia

Kristjansson E 2004 Reliability of ultrasonography for the cervical multifidus muscle in asymptomatic and symptomatic subjects. Manual Therapy 9:83-88

Lee D G 2003 The thorax; an integrated approach, 2nd edn. Diane G. Lee Physiotherapist Corp, White Rock, British Columbia

Lee D G 2004 The pelvic girdle; an approach to the examination and treatment of the lumbo-pelvic-hip region, 3rd edn. Churchill Livingstone, Edinburgh

Luft A R, Buitrago M M 2005 Stages of motor skill learning. Molecular Neurobiology 32(3):205-216

MacDonald D, Moseley G L, Hodges P W 2004 The function of the lumbar multifidus in unilateral low back pain. In: Proceedings of the 5th interdisciplinary world congress on low back and pelvic pain, Melbourne, Australia, p 329

Martan A, Masata J, Halaska M et al 2002 Ultrasound imaging of paravaginal defects in women with stress incontinence before and after paravaginal defect repair. Ultrasound in Obstetrics & Gynecology 19:496-500

McGill S 2002 Low back disorders – evidence-based prevention and rehabilitation. Human Kinetics, Canada

McMeeken J M, Beith I D, Newhan D J et al 2004 The relationship between EMG and changes in thickness of transversus abdominis. Clinical Biomechanics 19:337-342

McKenzie D, Gandevia S 1994 Dynamic changes in the zone of apposition and diaphragm length during maximal respiratory efforts. Thorax 49:634-638

Mens J M A, Vleeming A, Snijders C J et al 2001 Validity and reliability of the active straight leg raise test in posterior pelvic pain since pregnancy. Spine 26(10):1167-1171

Meyer S, De Grandi P, Schreyer A et al 1996 The assessment of bladder neck position and mobility in continent mullipara, multipara, forceps delivered and incontinent women using perineal ultrasound: A future office procedure? International Urogynecology Journal 7:138-146

Michlovitz S L 1990 Thermal agents in rehabilitation, 2nd edn. F A Davis, Philadelphia

Miller D L, Quddus J 2000 Diagnostic ultrasound activation of contrast agent gas bodies induces capillary rupture in mice. Proceedings of the National Academy of Science 97:10179-10184

Misuri G, Colagrande S, Gorini M et al 1997 In vivo ultrasound assessment of respiratory function of abdominal muscles in normal subjects. European Respiratory Journal 10:2861-2867

Moseley L G, Hodges P W, Gandevia S C 2002 Deep and superficial fibers of the lumbar multifidus muscle are differentially active during voluntary arm movements. Spine 27(2):E29-E36

Moseley L G 2003 A pain neuromatrix approach to patients with chronic pain. Manual Therapy 8(3):130-140

Murphy C, Sherburn M, Allen T 2002 Investigation of transabdominal diagnostic ultrasound as a clinical tool and outcome measure in the conservative management of pelvic floor muscle dysfunction. In: Proceedings of the international continence society meeting, Heidelberg, Abstract 129:61

Ng J K F, Kippers V, Richardson C A 1998 Muscle fiber orientation of abdominal muscles and suggested surface EMG electrode positions. Electromyography and Clinical Neurophysiology 38:51-58

Ng J K F, Richardson C A, Parnianpour M et al 2002 EMG activity of trunk muscles and torque output during isometric axial rotation exertion: a comparison between back pain patients and matched controls. Journal of Orthopaedic Research 20:112-121

Nguyen J K, Hall C D, Taber E et al 2000 Sonographic diagnosis of paravaginal defects: A standardization of technique. International Urogynecology Journal 11:341-345

Ninane V, Rypens F, Yernault J C et al 1992 Abdominal muscle use during breathing in patients with chronic airflow obstruction. American Review of Respiratory Disease 146:16-21

Nyborg W L 2001 Biological effects of ultrasound: development of safety guidelines. Part II: general review. Ultrasound in Medicine & Biology 27(3):301-333

Nyborg W L 2002 Safety of medical diagnostic ultrasound. Seminars in Ultrasound, CT and MRI 23(5):377-386

Ostrzenski A, Osborne N G 1998 Ultrasonography as a screening tool for paravaginal defects in women with stress incontinence: A pilot study. International Urogynecology Journal 9:105-199

O'Sullivan P B, Twomey L T, Allison G T 1997 Evaluation of specific stabilizing exercise in the treatment of chronic low back pain with radiologic diagnosis of spondylolysis or spondylolisthesis. Spine 22: 2959-2967

O'Sullivan P B 2000 Lumbar segmental "instability": clinical presentation and specific stabilizing exercise management. Manual Therapy 5(1):2-12

O'Sullivan P B, Beales D J, Beetham J A et al 2002 Altered motor control strategies in subjects with sacro-iliac joint pain during the active straight leg raise test. Spine 27(1):E1-E8

O'Sullivan P B 2005 Diagnosis and classification of chronic low back pain disorders: Maladaptive movement and motor control impairments as underlying mechanism. Manual Therapy 10(4):242-255

Panjabi M 1992 The stabilizing system of the spine. Part I: function, dysfunction, adaptation, and enhancement. Journal of Spinal Disorders 5(4):383-389

Peschers U, Schaer G, Anthuber C et al 1996 Changes in vesical neck mobility following vaginal delivery. Obstetrics and Gynaecology 88: 1001-1006

Peschers U M, Vodusek D B, Fanger G et al 2001a Pelvic muscle activity in nulliparous volunteers. Neurourology and Urodynamics 20:269-275

Peschers U M, Gingelmaier A, Jundt K et al 2001b Evaluation of pelvic floor muscle strength using four different techniques. International Urogynecology Journal 12:27-30

Pranathi Reddy A, DeLancey J O L, Zwica L, Ashton-Miller J A 2001 On-screen vector-based ultrasound assessment of vesical neck movement. American Journal of Obstetrics and Gynecology 185:65-70

Rankin G, Stokes M 1998 Reliability of assessment tools in rehabilitation: an illustration of appropriate statistical analyses. Clinical Rehabilitation 12:187-199

Rankin G, Stokes M, Newham D J 2005 Size and shape of the posterior neck muscles measured by ultrasound imaging: values in males and females of different ages. Manual Therapy 10:108-115

Rath A M, Attali P, Dumas J L et al 1996 The abdominal linea alba: an anatomo-radiologic and biomechanical study. Surgical and Radiologic Anatomy 18:281-288

Rettenbacher T, Hollerweger A, Macheiner P et al 2001 Abdominal wall hernias: Cross sectional imaging signs of incarceration determined with sonography. American Journal of Radiology 177:1061-1066

Richardson C A, Hodges P W, Hides J A 2004 Therapeutic exercise for spinal segmental stabilization: A motor control approach for the treatment and prevention of low back pain, 2nd edn. Churchill Livingstone, Edinburgh

Rosenbaum D A, Carlson R A, Gilmore R O 2001 Acquisition of intellectual and perceptual motor skills. Annual Reviews in Psychology 52:453-470

Salmoni A W, Schmidt R A, Walter C B 1984 Knowledge of results and motor learning: A review and critical reappraisal. Psychological Bulletin 95(3):355-386

Sapsford R R, Bullock-Saxton J, Markwell S 1998 Women's health: a textbook for physiotherapists. W B Saunders, London

Sapsford R R, Hodges P W, Richardson C A et al 2001 Co-activation of the abdominal and pelvic floor muscles during voluntary exercises. Neurourology and Urodynamics 20:31-42

Sapsford R R, Hodges P W 2001 Contraction of the pelvic floor muscles during abdominal maneuvers. Archives of Physical Medicine and Rehabilitation 82:1081-1088

Sapsford R R 2004 Rehabilitation of pelvic floor muscles utilizing trunk stabilization. Manual Therapy 9:3-12

Saunders S W, Rath D, Hodges P W 2004 Postural and respiratory activation of the trunk muscles changes with mode and speed of locomotion. Gait and Posture 20(3):280-290 (PMID: 15531175)

Schaer G N, Koechli O R, Schuessler B et al 1995 Perineal ultrasound for evaluating the bladder neck in urinary stress incontinence. Obstetrics and Gynecology 85:220-224

Schaer G N, Perucchini D, Munz E et al 1999 Sonographic evaluation of the bladder neck in continent and stress-incontinent women. Obstetrics and Gynecology 93(3):412-416

Sheppard S 1996 Case study: The role of transversus abdominis in post partum correction of gross divarication recti. Manual Therapy 1(4):214-216

Sherburn M, Murphy C A, Carroll S et al 2005 Investigation of transabdominal real-time ultrasound to visualize the muscles of the pelvic floor. The Australian Journal of Physiotherapy 51:167-170

Shiffrin R M, Schneider W 1977 Controlled and automatic human information processing: II Perceptual learning, automatic attending and a general theory. Psychological Review 84:127-190

Shirado O, Ito T, Kaneda K, Strax T E 1995 Flexion-relaxation phenomenon in the back muscles. A comparative study between healthy subjects and patients with chronic low back pain. American Journal of Physical Medicine and Rehabilitation 74(2):139-144

Stokes M, Hides J, Nassiri D K 1997 Musculoskeletal ultrasound imaging: diagnostic and treatment aid in rehabilitation. Physical Therapy Review 2:73-92

Stokes M, Rankin G, Newham D J 2005 Ultrasound imaging of lumbar multifidus muscle: normal reference ranges for measurements and practical guidance on the technique. Manual Therapy 10:116-126

Strobel K, Holder J, Meyer D C et al 2005 Fatty atrophy of supraspinatus and infraspinatus muscles: accuracy of ultrasound. Radiology 237:584-589

Strohl K P, Mead J, Banzett R B et al 1981 Regional differences in abdominal muscle activity during various maneuvers in humans. Journal of Applied Physiology 51(6):1471-1476

Stuge B, Laerum E, Kirkesola G et al 2004 The efficacy of a treatment program focusing on specific stabilizing exercises for pelvic girdle pain after pregnancy. Spine 29(4):351-359

Stuge B, Mørkved S, Dahl H H et al 2006a Abdominal and pelvic floor muscle function in women with and without long lasting pelvic girdle pain. Manual Therapy (in press)

Stuge B, Holm I, Vøllestad N 2006b To treat or not to treat postpartum pelvic girdle pain with stabilizing exercises. Manual Therapy Jan 6; (Epub ahead of press)

Teyhen D, Miltenberger C E, Deiters H M et al 2005 The use of ultrasound imaging of the abdominal drawing in maneuver in subjects with low back pain. Journal of Orthopaedic & Sports Physical Therapy 35(6):346-355

Thompson J A, O'Sullivan P B 2003 Levator plate movement during voluntary pelvic floor muscle contraction in subjects with incontinence and prolapse: a cross-sectional study and review. International Urogynecology Journal 14:84-88

Thompson J A, O'Sullivan P B, Briffa K et al 2005 Assessment of pelvic floor movement using transabdominal and transperineal ultrasound. International Urogynecology Journal 16:285-292

Thompson J A, O'Sullivan P B, Briffa K et al 2006a Differences in muscle activation patterns during pelvic floor muscle contraction and valsalva manoeuvre. Neurourology and Urodynamics 25(2):148-155

Thompson J A, O'Sullivan P B, Briffa N K, Neumann P 2006b Altered muscle activation patterns in symptomatic women during pelvic floor muscle contraction and valsalva manoeuvre. Neurology and Urodynamics 25(3):268-276

Thorn B E 2004 Cognitive therapy for chronic pain. The Guildford Press, New York

Toranto R 1990 The relief of low back pain with the WARP abdominoplasty: a preliminary report. Plastic and Reconstructive Surgery 85:545-555

Tsubahara A, Chino N, Akaboshi K et al 1995 Age related changes of water and fat content in muscles estimated by magnetic resonance imaging. Disability and Rehabilitation 17:298-304

Ueki J, De Bruin P F, Pride N B 1995 In vivo assessment of diaphragm contraction by ultrasound in normal subjects. Thorax 50:1157-1161

Urquhart D M, Barker P J, Hodges P W et al 2005 Regional morphology of the transversus abdominis and obliqus internus and externus abdominis muscles. Clinical Biomechanics 20:233-241

van Dieën J H, Selen L P J, Cholewicki J 2003 Trunk muscle activation in low-back pain patients, an analysis of the literature. Journal of Electromyography and Kinesiology 13:333-351

Van Holsbeeck M T, Introcas J H 2001 Musculoskeletal ultrasound. Mosby, St. Louis

van Uchelen J H, Kon M, Werker P M N 2001 The long term durability of placation of the anterior rectus sheath assessed by ultrasonography. Plastic and Reconstructive Surgery 197:1578-1584

Vleeming A, Snijders C J, Stoeckart R et al 1997 The role of the sacroiliac joints in coupling between spine, pelvis, legs and arms. In: Vleeming A, Mooney V, Dorman T, Snijders C, Stoeckart R (eds) Movement, stability and low back pain; the essential role of the pelvis. Churchill Livingstone, New York, p 53-71

Walz P H, Bertermann H 1990 Ultrasound examination of bladder and prostate. Urologia Internationalis 45:217-230

Watanabe K, Miyamoto K, Masuda T et al 2004 Use of ultrasonography to evaluate thickness of the erector spinae muscle in maximum flexion and extension of the lumbar spine. Spine 29(13):1472-1477

WCPT 1999 World confederation for physical therapy, declaration of principle and position statements; description of physical therapy – position statement. Online. Available: http://www.wcpt.org, May 1999

Whittaker J L 2004a Abdominal ultrasound imaging of pelvic floor muscle function in individuals with low back pain. Journal of Manual and Manipulative Therapy 12(1):44-49

Whittaker J L 2004b Real-time ultrasound analysis of local system function. In: Lee D G The pelvic girdle; An approach to the examination and treatment of the lumbopelvic-hip region, 3rd edn. Churchill Livingstone, Edinburgh, p 120-129

Whittaker J L 2004c Recommendations for the implementation of real time ultrasound imaging in physical therapy practice. The final report of a College of Physical Therapists of British Columbia real time ultrasound imaging ad hoc committee

Whittaker J L 2005 Ultrasound imaging characteristics of individuals with pelvic instability and concurrent respiratory dysfunction. In: Proceedings of the 2nd International Conference on Movement Dysfunction, Pain and Performance: Evidence and Effect, Edinburgh, UK

WHO 1982 Environmental health criteria 22: Ultrasound. World Health Organization, Geneva

WHO 1989 Ultrasound. In: Nonionizing radiation protection, 2nd edn. World Health Organization, Geneva

Wijma J, Tinga D J, Visser G H A 1991 Perineal ultrasonography in women with stress incontinence and control: the role of the pelvic floor muscles. Gynecologic and Obstetric Investigation 32:176-179

Williams P L 1995 Gray's anatomy; The anatomical basis of medicine and surgery, 38th edn. Churchill Livingstone, New York

Wiss R 2002 EDE – Emergency department echo. The essentials of emergency department ultrasound. Course notes

Zedka M, Prochazka A, Knight B et al 1999 Voluntary and reflex control of human back muscles during induced pain. Journal of Physiology (London) 520:591-604

APPENDIX A
Outline – lumbopelvic USI assessment

BLADDER AND PELVIC FLOOR RESTING STATE		
USI – QUALITATIVE ANALYSIS	TRANSVERSE	SAGITTAL
Presence of respiratory motion of bladder at rest (Y/N)		
Shape and symmetry of the bladder at rest (describe)		
Relationship of the bladder to the pelvic floor (height)		

BLADDER AND PELVIC FLOOR WITH A LOADING TASK (e.g. ASLR)		
USI – QUALITATIVE ANALYSIS	TRANSVERSE	SAGITTAL
Caudodorsal motion of bladder with task (Y/N)		
Dorsal motion of bladder with task (Y/N)		
Lateral shift or rotation of bladder with task (direction)		
Observable PFM contraction during task (Y/N)		
Decrease in shape of the bladder (Y/N)		

USI – QUANTITATIVE ANALYSIS	TRANSVERSE	SAGITTAL
Caudodorsal distance with task		
Dorsal distance with task		
Angle with respect to image horizontal		
Lateral distance from midline with task		

PREFERENTIAL ACTIVATION OF THE PFM

USI – QUALITATIVE ANALYSIS	TRANSVERSE	SAGITTAL
Caudal encroachment of bladder with contraction (Y/N)		
Abdominal encroachment of bladder with contraction (Y/N)		
Caudodorsal motion of bladder with contraction (Y/N)		
Cranioventral motion of bladder with contraction (Y/N)		
Decrease in shape of the bladder (Y/N)		
Observable relaxation of the PFM after the contraction (Y/N)		

USI – QUALITATIVE ANALYSIS	TRANSVERSE	SAGITTAL
Caudodorsal distance with task		
Cranioventral distance with task		
Angle with respect to image horizontal		

ABDOMINAL WALL RESTING STATE

USI – QUALITATIVE ANALYSIS	LEFT	RIGHT
Integrity of the linea alba (quality of architectural delineation)		
Resting respiratory modulation (TrA, IO or both) (a+ = >20%)		
TrA resting state (normal, hypertonic)		
IO resting state (normal, hypertonic)		
Quality of muscle (RA, EO, IO, TrA) (hypoechoic = <50%, hyperechoic = >50%)		
Distance from the midline to the linea semilunaris		

USI QUANTITATIVE ANALYSIS – RESPIRATION	INSPIRATION		EXPIRATION		% CHANGE	
	LEFT	RIGHT	LEFT	RIGHT	LEFT	RIGHT
TA – depth						
IO – depth						

ABDOMINAL WALL WITH A LOADING TASK, (e.g. ASLR)

USI – QUALITATIVE ANALYSIS	LEFT	RIGHT
Width of the linea alba (static, ↑ or ↓ in width)		
TrA co-activation throughout task (Y/N)		
Altered TrA co-activation (absent, irregular or excessive)		
IO co-activation throughout task (Y/N)		
Altered IO co-activation (absent, irregular or excessive)		
TrA relaxation after task (Y/N)		
IO relaxation after task (Y/N)		

USI – QUANTITATIVE ANALYSIS	RESTING		CONTRACTED		% CHANGE	
	LEFT	RIGHT	LEFT	RIGHT	LEFT	RIGHT
TrA – depth						
TrA – length						
IO – depth						

ABDOMINAL WALL WITH PREFERENTIAL ACTIVATION OF TrA

USI – QUALITATIVE ANALYSIS	LEFT	RIGHT
Effect of TrA on linea alba (static, ↑ or ↓ in width)		
Lateral slide of TrA under IO (Y/N)		
Lateral corset of TrA (Y/N)		
Lateral corset of IO (Y/N)		
↑ TrA girth with activation (Y/N)		
↑ IO girth with activation (Y/N)		
TrA Relaxation after contraction (Y/N)		
IO Relaxation after contraction (Y/N)		

USI QUANTITATIVE ANALYSIS	RESTING		CONTRACTED		% CHANGE	
	LEFT	RIGHT	LEFT	RIGHT	LEFT	RIGHT
TrA – depth						
TrA – length						
IO – depth						
Midline to linea semilunaris – width						
Linea alba – width						

MULTIFIDUS RESTING STATE

USI – QUALITATIVE ANALYSIS	LEFT	RIGHT
Resting shape – level (symmetrical, round, oval or triangular)		
Resting size – level (symmetrical, asymmetrical)		
Quality of muscle (MF) (hypoechoic = <50%, hyperechoic = >50%)		

MULTIFIDUS WITH A LOADING TASK (e.g. prone or lateral leg lift)

USI – QUALITATIVE ANALYSIS	LEFT	RIGHT
MF co-activation throughout task (Y/N)		
Altered MF co-activation (absent, irregular or excessive)		
MF relaxation after task (Y/N)		

PREFERENTIAL ACTIVATION OF MULTIFIDUS

USI – QUALITATIVE ANALYSIS	LEFT	RIGHT
Observed increase in dMF depth – level (Y/N)		
Observed increase in sMF depth – level (Y/N)		
Anterior motion of spinal column (segmental vs. multi-segmental)		
Speed of contraction (tonic vs. phasic)		
MF relaxation after task (Y/N)		

USI – QUANTITATIVE ANALYSIS	WIDTH				DEPTH				% CHANGE			
	RESTING		CONTRACTION		RESTING		CONTRACTION		WIDTH		DEPTH	
	L	R	L	R	L	R	L	R	L	R	L	R
L2												
L3												
L4												
L5												
S1												

APPENDIX B
Outline of the minimum requirements for an ultrasound imaging accreditation process for rehabilitation professionals

A primary concern regarding the use of ultrasound imaging (USI) by physiotherapists and other rehabilitation professionals is the need for standardized training. As the clinical use of ultrasound imaging for the assessment and treatment of neuromuscular control is in its infancy, it is imperative that the credentialing mechanisms that are being considered are rigorous, and reflect the highest standards of quality control. As such this brief appendix is devoted to topics related to the format, curriculum and instruction of such a process.

The clinical application of USI involves three steps: image generation (the ability to generate a clear image of the structure(s) that is of interest), image recognition (the ability to orientate oneself to the two-dimensional nature of an ultrasound image), and image interpretation (the ability to interpret both static and dynamic images). Consequently, these three processes and the information required for their development serve as the foundation of all training programmes. Although there is some fundamental information that is generic (principle of ultrasound wave propagation, instrumentation, etc.), the material covered varies substantially depending on the intent of the examiner. For example, traditional medical imaging applications involve the generation and interpretation of a very wide range of tissues. As such, medical sonographers and radiologists require extensive training in the recognition of the diverse aspect of normal and abnormal anatomy. Alternatively, in the rehabilitation field the interest is primarily in viewing muscle (and perhaps nerve), both in its static form and during a dynamic event (neuromuscular control). Although rehabilitation professionals share in their requirement for certain fundamental information, their training presents a unique challenge. Specifically, there is a need for a very diverse theoretical background (regional anatomy and motor control), a requirement of a basic level of clinical expertise (USI is not intended as a stand-alone assessment or treatment tool, rather is incorporated alongside existing clinical skills), and the challenge of delivering postgraduate education on a topic that requires repeated practical exposure.

In 2004 an ad hoc committee was established by the College of Physical Therapists of British Columbia, Canada to investigate and provide recommendations regarding the implementation of USI in physiotherapy practice. This committee addressed several issues; however, one of its primary purposes was to address the structure and curriculum of an accreditation process for its members. The committee took into consideration the accreditation processes of other health-related professional associations, as well as expert opinion; it deliberated over various formats for delivery, ranging from correspondence and self-study, to course study, as well as residency. Ultimately, the recommendations for *minimum* requirements (which are presented here) were a process that involved both self- and course study followed by practical evaluation.

SUGGESTED CURRICULUM

The format of the suggested accreditation process (self-study followed by an 18-hour practical course) is intended to provide physiotherapists with the *minimum* basic knowledge and skills required for the safe integration of USI into clinical practice. As USI has the potential to be applied to many muscle groups throughout the body, it is accepted that the preliminary list of scans included in the course curriculum will expand in time. Although USI of muscle groups is generic in some regards, all scans require very specific anatomical and neurophysiological knowledge. This accreditation process is aimed at providing only the generic principles on which clinicians can base further training.

Prerequisite reading (to be completed prior to course study)

I. Students are expected to read selected articles from peer-reviewed journals and texts that cover topics such as the nature and propagation of ultrasound waves and ultrasound instrumentation, as well as the technical, safety and practical aspects of USI.

II. Students are expected to demonstrate sound knowledge of the neuromuscular mechanisms of the lumbopelvic region with regard to postural control of the trunk, respiration and continence, both in health and during dysfunction. It is likely that this requirement will be fulfilled through both preliminary self-study and previous course work.

In an attempt to ensure that this material has been thoroughly covered prior to entering into course work a remote closed-book, invigilated exam could be administered.

Course outline

This suggested curriculum contains material that can be covered in 18 hours. However, it can also serve as an outline for more comprehensive instruction.

I. Introduction

a. Outline the goals and objectives of the course.

b. Define the differences between medical musculoskeletal USI (diagnosis of ligament, tendon, muscle structural pathology by radiologists and sonographers) and rehabilitative musculoskeletal USI (applications that result in a physical diagnosis of the size or movement characteristics of muscles and/or nerves in relation to adjacent structures, or involve the use of USI as a biofeedback tool by physiotherapists).

   i. History of the use of USI in physiotherapy.

   ii. Scope of practice issues, including a model for communication with other health care professionals who employ USI.

   iii. Current clinical uses of USI in physiotherapy (see the list of current physiotherapy USI applications below).

   iv. Limitations to the use of USI in physiotherapy.

II. Physics of sound

a. The nature of ultrasound waves, including a discussion on topics such as amplitude, frequency, wavelength, intensity, power, propagation speed, pulsed ultrasound, attenuation, absorption, refection, scattering, resolution and penetration.

b. The nature of an ultrasound echo, including a discussion on topics such as the angle of incidence, impedance, refraction and the difference between a reflector or a scatterer, as well as the effects of different tissue densities.

III. Instrumentation

a. Transducers (construction, operation, focusing, types of arrays and their uses, resolution).

b. Imaging instruments (components and their function as well as brightness and motion display modes).

IV. Safety and risk of harm issues

a. Thermal considerations.

b. Mechanical considerations.

c. ALARA (as low as reasonably achievable) principle, including a discussion on how to minimize power output in favour of higher gain settings.

d. Identification of specific individuals or situations at higher risk of harm.

e. Discussion of a generic plan of action and model of communication for incidences in which unusual structures are identified while performing an USI assessment of motor control.

V. Understanding static ultrasound images

a. 2-D representations of 3-D anatomical structures.

b. 2-D planes of view and motion.

c. Image modulation (near, far and total gain, brightness, focal zones).

d. Artefact (general definition, as well as the basic types, their causes and implications).

e. Specific tissue identification (bone, fascia, fluid, muscle, tendon etc.).

VI. Indications for the use of USI in physiotherapy

a. Identification of individuals with neuromuscular dysfunction (particularly in the vertebral column).

b. A review of contemporary approaches regarding neuromuscular control of the spine.

c. A review of the literature surrounding the topic of spinal postural control, including a review of the anatomy and activation studies of the muscles responsible for postural control, respiration and continence.

VII. USI in the lumbopelvic region – assessment

a. Overview of the functions of ultrasound instrumentation (transducer specifics, probe orientation, control buttons etc.).

b. Didactic sessions:

   i. Instruction in the generation of ultrasound images of the abdominal wall, lumbar spine and pelvic floor.

   ii. Presentation of various normal and abnormal images, both as static images and real-time video clips.

   iii. Interpretation of various normal and abnormal images from the abdominal wall, lumbar spine and pelvic floor.

   iv. Demonstration of the uses of USI for measuring the architectural features of muscle (depth, width, cross-sectional area).

c. Practical sessions:

   i. Demonstration of techniques to generate images of the abdominal wall, lumbar spine, and pelvic floor.

   ii. Practice aimed at generating images of the abdominal wall, lumbar spine and pelvic floor.

   iii. Practice aimed at interpreting muscle and fascial echogenicity (limitations) and architectural delineations.

   iv. Practice aimed at interpreting images of load transfer through the lumbopelvic region, abdominal wall, lumbar spine and pelvic floor in both normal and abnormal cohorts.

   v. Practice aimed at interpreting images of preferential activation of specific deep system muscles (e.g. transversus abdominis, the deep segmental fibres of lumbar multifidus and the pelvic floor muscles), as well as their influence on the fascial tissue into which they attach.

   vi. Practice aimed at measuring the architectural features of muscle.

At present, the majority of USI applications of interest to the rehabilitation professional centre around the lumbopelvic region. However, as USI has the potential to be applied to many muscle groups throughout the body it is expected that the preliminary list of scans included in this curriculum will expand. For the purpose of this suggested curriculum, and in keeping with the topic of this text, the area of instruction is the lumbopelvic region. However, this section could easily be replaced or augmented with scans involving the thoracic and cervical spines, as well as the diaphragm.

VIII. Practical evaluation and conclusion

a. Final evaluation will involve the performance of a set number of scans (including at least four different muscle groups) in which the candidate generates and then presents an interpretation of their findings to the instructor. All but two of the scans must be dynamic in nature, with the two static scans involving measurement of an architectural parameter of a muscle (one linear and one circumferential).

LIST OF CURRENT PHYSIOTHERAPY USI APPLICATIONS

This generic list of imaging applications encompasses those reported within the existing literature as well as those common to current clinical practice.

I. The abdominal wall, including midline and lateral aspects – for the purpose of speculating on and measuring midline abdominal fascial defects, as well as for commenting upon the behaviour, and measuring the architectural changes, of the abdominal muscles (rectus abdominis, internal oblique, external oblique and transversus abdominis) during a variety of efforts (Misuri et al 1997, Richardson et al 2004, Whittaker 2004b).

II. The pelvic floor through an abdominal view – for the purpose of determining positional bladder stability during tests of load transfer through the lumbopelvic region (O'Sullivan et al 2002), as well as for viewing and measuring the impact of a pelvic floor muscle contraction on the bladder (Murphy et al 2002, Thompson & O'Sullivan 2003, Whittaker 2004a, Sherburn et al 2005, Thompson et al 2005).

III. The pelvic floor muscles through a perineal view – for the purpose of determining positional bladder stability during tests of load transfer through the lumbopelvic region, as well as for viewing and measuring the impact of a pelvic floor muscle contraction on the bladder, and urethrovesical neck (Schaer et al 1999, Dietz et al 2001, Peschers et al 2001b).

IV. The spinal musculature in the lumbopelvic, thoracic and cervical spine – for the purpose of viewing and measuring the architectural changes of these muscles during a contraction. This may include the multifidus and other deep spinal muscles, the erector spinae at various spinal levels (Hides et al 1992, Coldron et al 2003, Kristjansson 2004, Watanabe et al 2004, Rankin et al 2005, Stokes et al 2005), as well as quadratus lumborum and psoas (Elliot et al 2004).

V. The diaphragm through a lateral thoracic view – for the purpose of viewing and measuring the architectural changes of the diaphragm during a contraction (Hodges et al 1997, Blaney 1999 et al).

SUGGESTED QUALIFICATIONS OF INSTRUCTORS

Ultimately, it is suggested that instructors and examiners of this material be individuals who have completed the accreditation process, who utilize the technology in their practice on a daily basis, and who have gone on to assist and co-instruct the curriculum under the instruction of a senior instructor. However, since most accreditation processes are in their infancy, and few such senior instructors exist, it is suggested that licensing boards initially identify individuals either within or outside their membership who have the expertise and experience to instruct as well as evaluate the curriculum, and appoint them as senior instructors.

APPENDIX C
The clinical application of USI in the treatment of lumbopelvic dysfunction: a case presentation

A 27-year-old male presented with complaints of pain and tightness in his right lower back and buttock, secondary to a fall onto this region while snowboarding three months earlier (**Fig. C.1**). The patient reported that his symptoms were aggravated with weight-bearing activities such as prolonged walking or standing, and that he had been unable to run or snowboard without pain since the incident. Non-weight-bearing positions provided some relief; however, there was a persistent aching sensation. The patient was allegedly otherwise healthy, and denied pharmaceutical management or the presence of any back, pelvic or hip symptoms prior to the incident. An x-ray of the pelvis and lumbar spine taken the day of the incident was reportedly normal. His initial Roland–Morris (RM) score was 17/24.

On observation there was considerable tone evident in the right thoracolumbar erector spinae, as well as a lordosis that extended from L3 to T8. The centre of gravity of the thorax was situated posterior to that of a posteriorly rotated pelvis, and the right femur was held in slight external rotation. On assessment of the gross movements of the region, asymmetry was detected with both forward (rotated to the right near full flexion with a pulling sensation in the right lower back and buttock) and backward bending (rotated left near full extension with an impingement sensation in the right lower back). Left side flexion was restricted and produced a pulling sensation in the right flank, low back and buttock, while

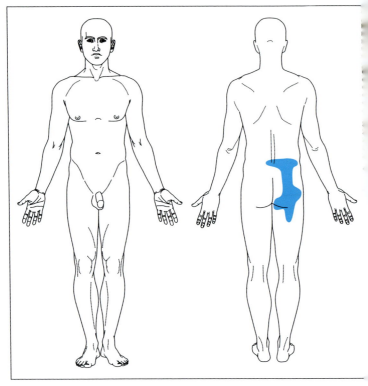

Figure C.1 Location of symptoms.

right side flexion was within normal limits, however, it resulted in a mild binding sensation in this same region.

Passive mobility testing of the sacroiliac joints (Lee 2004) detected increased stiffness in the vertical component of right joint compared with the left, with the end-feel suggestive of a joint fixation. Passive intervertebral motion testing (PIVM) in the lumbar spine revealed irritability to posterior inferior motion of the right L5 zygapophyseal articular surface on S1. Furthermore, the passive accessory intervertebral motions (PAIVM) at this segment were found to be more abrupt than the left, and the end-feel indicated restriction due to increased muscle tone. Mobility testing of the right hip detected a decrease in flexion and internal rotation. Tests of hip joint accessory motion (PAM) indicated an articular restriction of flexion (anterior impingement) and an extra-articular restriction of internal rotation (tone in the external rotator muscles). Due to the hypomobility detected at the sacroiliac, lumbar and hip joints, stability tests were not indicated.

When the patient was asked to stand on his left leg and bring his right hip into flexion (the non-weight-bearing one-leg standing test (NWB OLS) (Hungerford et al 2004, Lee 2004) there was a loss of posterior rotation of the right innominate relative to the sacrum. When the patient stood on the right leg and flexed the left hip (the standing load transfer or the weight-bearing one-leg standing test (WB OLS) he had difficulty in maintaining control over the support leg. During the active straight leg raise test (ASLR) (Mens et al 2001, Lee 2004) the patient found it more difficult to lift the right leg up off the bed, and the addition of further compression to the pelvis (particularly if it was applied posteriorly) increased his pain, and decreased his ability to lift the leg.

Nerve conduction tests were normal, while nerve mobility tests indicated a slight decrease in the mobility of the right sciatic nerve (detected at the end-range of a slump test) (Butler 2000). Hypertonicity of the right iliocostalis lumborum, piriformis, ischiococcygeus, small external rotators of the hip, internal oblique (IO) and biceps femoris was detected through palpation. Due to the presence of joint and neuromeningeal hypomobility, and the considerable hypertonicity in the regional muscles, assessment of the deep muscle system was not performed.

Following completion of the assessment a high-velocity, low-amplitude gap (manipulation) was performed on the right sacroiliac joint, followed by dry needling directed at the right iliocostalis lumborum, piriformis, ischiococcygeus, small external rotators of the hip and biceps femoris (Lee 2004). On immediate reassessment the right sacroiliac joint demonstrated the following:

- There was improved posterior rotation of the right innominate relative to the sacrum during the NWB phase of the OLS test, but failure to maintain a self-locked position (relative nutation) with the WB phase of the OLS test (the innominate rotated anterior relative to the sacrum).

- The right ASLR also showed improvement, although the leg appeared heavier and remained more difficult to lift than the left. The ability to lift the right leg improved when compression was provided across the inferior aspect of the pelvis (a force meant to mimic the contribution of the PFM to force closure of the pelvis) in combination with lengthening of the right thoracolumbar region (Lee 2004).

- Mobility testing indicated a decrease in stiffness in the vertical plane and, the subsequent passive stability test suggested a mild insufficiency in the passive elements that control the vertical glide at this joint.

- Nerve mobility testing continued to indicate decreased freedom of the right sciatic nerve.

The conclusion at the end of the first session was that the patient had presented with a fixation of the right sacroiliac joint in combination with associated hypertonicity secondary to trauma. After the fixation was addressed it was apparent that the right sacroiliac joint was functionally unstable secondary to both passive (ligamentous and joint capsule) and active (muscles) insufficiencies (Panjabi 1992, Lee 2004). In particular, it appeared that the active insufficiency was with respect to the inferior aspect of the pelvis. Education was provided to this end and the patient was shown how to self-release the hypertonicity in his right buttock region by using a soft racquet ball, as well as how to mobilize the right sciatic nerve (Butler 2000). The patient was then advised to return in approximately one week.

The patient reported a considerable decrease in his symptoms at the second session but that he was still having difficulty standing or walking for any length of time (RM = 12/24). He had not performed the self-release exercises aimed at the hypertonic buttock muscles; however, he had been diligent in his nerve mobilizations. Assessment findings were similar to what had been seen post treatment in the first session:

- When performing a right ASLR the patient continued to benefit from compression to the inferior aspect of the pelvis but had a slight increase in his pain with posterior compression aimed at approximating the posterior superior iliac spines (PSIS). These findings indicated a deficiency in the compression of the inferior aspect and either intolerance to, or excessive compression of the posterosuperior aspect of the pelvis.

- The hypertonicity in the right IO, iliocostalis lumborum, piriformis, ischiococcygeus and small external rotators of the hip persisted.

- Nerve mobility testing had improved only slightly.

Treatment proceeded with further dry needling to the right iliocostalis lumborum, superficial multifidus, piriformis, ischiococcygeus and small external rotators of the hip (Lee 2004). Once the tone in these muscles was diminished, the patient was encouraged to relax his thoracolumbar lordosis, posterior pelvic tilt and buttock-clenching in a crook lie position. Doing so helped to establish a more neutral spinal posture, decompressed the right L5S1 zygapophyseal joint and allowed space for the right femoral head to begin to reseat itself within the acetabulum.

Once the sacroiliac and lumbar zygapophyseal joints were decompressed, the hypertonicity of the surrounding muscles minimized and the spine relaxed into a neutral posture, a sagittal ultrasound image of the bladder was generated through the abdomen (**Figs 2.10, 2.11a, b**) and the ASLR test was repeated (**Fig. 3.17a, b**). Although the bladder remained virtually stationary during the ASLR test on the left, it demonstrated an obvious descent when the right leg was lifted. This finding suggested the use of a suboptimal motor control strategy involving a straining-type activation (excessive response) of the diaphragm and abdominal wall muscles, resulting in a downwardly directed increase in IAP which overwhelmed the ability of the pelvic floor to support the bladder (O'Sullivan et al 2002). In an attempt to ascertain the status of the PFM the ultrasound probe was rotated to the transverse plane (**Figs 2.12, 2.13a, b**), and the patient's ability to preferentially activate these muscles was evaluated. The resulting ultrasound image demonstrated a straining or valsalva activation pattern associated with a posterior pelvic tilt (**Fig. 3.22b**). No encroachment of the gluteal border of the bladder wall by the PFM was observed.

Through education (particularly of the orientation and anatomy of the PFM), imagery and use of USI, preferential activation of the PFM was achieved over a short period of time. The isolated contraction was then practised in conjunction with USI feedback in an attempt to solidify the internal awareness of the contraction so that it could be practised at home. The patient was given cues to focus on, independent of the ultrasound image, that would help him to identify an inaccurate contraction. This included the behaviour of his abdominal wall (palpable contraction of his obliques) and breath holding. Although the isolated contraction resulted in moderate encroachment of the bladder wall, it fatigued quickly, and the patient had a tendency to revert to a straining strategy with an increase in effort. However, when the ASLR and vertical stability test of the sacroiliac joint were retested, while the isolated PFM contraction was held (confirmed by USI), both tests normalized (e.g. the right leg became easier to lift than previously and the bladder remained stationary when imaged, while the stiffness of the vertical glide was greater and more consistent in relation to the left side).

The patient's instructions for home at the conclusion of the second session were to continue releasing any persisting hypertonicity in the region through trigger-point work, as well as continued sciatic nerve mobilization. In addition, the patient was encouraged to spend time relaxing into a neutral spinal position followed by isolated contractions of the PFM.

On the third visit the patient continued to report a decrease in his symptoms as well as a slight improvement in his tolerance of vertical loading (walking and standing) (RM = 9/24). On reassessment the findings showed:

- The right ASLR was positive and he continued to benefit from compression to the inferior aspect of the right innominate or conscious activation of the PFM, as well as decompression of the right thoracolumbar region. Furthermore, there was no increase in pain associated with posterior compression which approximated the PSISs.

- The hypertonicity in the right iliocostalis lumborum, piriformis, ischiococcygeus and small external rotators of the hip had improved significantly. However, some excessive tone remained in the right IO.

- Nerve mobility testing had normalized.

The goals for this session were to address any remaining hypertonicity, reinforce relaxing into a neutral spinal position and assess the coordination of the deep muscle system of the region. The patient was anxious to confirm the accuracy of his PFM contraction, so the session began with a reassessment of motor control augmented by USI. Transverse imaging of the bladder confirmed his ability to contract his PFM, but that the contraction was followed immediately by a descent of the bladder. This indicated that although there was momentary preferential activation of the PFM, this was almost instantaneously accompanied with a straining effort which was detected as bladder descent. Consequently, the initial focus of the session was spent teaching the patient how to eliminate the second (straining) stage of the effort and perfect the subtlety of PFM isolation.

Once the patient could confidently isolate his PFM, both with feedback from USI, as well as performing it with his eyes closed, the ultrasound probe was moved to the lateral abdominal wall so as to visualize the coordination between the PFM, TrA, and respiration (**Figs 2.2, 2.3a, b**) (Sapsford et al 2001). When the patient contracted his PFM an associated co-contraction of the left TrA was detected (**Fig. 3.5a, b**); however, a simultaneous contraction of both the TrA and IO was seen on the right (**Fig. 3.7a**). Furthermore, resting respiratory modulation (increase in depth, and decrease in length >20% associated with expiration) of both the right TrA and IO was observed (**Fig. 3.2a, b**). As a modulated contraction of TrA (or the IO) corresponding to resting expiration is an indicator of dysfunction (an increase in chemical drive or the elastic loading due to joint fixation, disease process or hypertonicity of the superficial muscles that attach to the thorax), further attempts to preferentially activate the right TrA would have been inappropriate (Whittaker 2005). Consequently, dry needling was administered to the trigger points in the right IO followed by breath work emphasizing lateral costal expansion and a passive expiratory phase equal in length to inspiration. At the completion of this the coordination of the PFM and TrA was reassessed, while maintaining the new respiratory strategy and a co-contraction of the right TrA was detected.

The patient was sent home with the goals of controlling the hypertonicity in his right IO through trigger point, respiratory and neutral spine work. He was to continue to practise the subtle PFM contraction, focusing on maintaining the new respiratory strategy, while attempting longer holds and changing postures (supine, sitting, standing etc.).

On the fourth visit the patient continued to report a decrease in his symptoms and an improvement in his tolerance of vertical loading (walking and standing) (RM 6/24). As he was having fewer symptoms he was anxious to return to recreational activities. On reassessment the findings showed:

- The right ASLR was improved; however, he continued to benefit slightly from lengthening of the right IO, indicating some residual hypertonus (Lee 2004).

- The right WB phase of the OLS test was normal; however, he still had a tendency to lock his hip into external rotation and drive his femoral head anterior as the length of time that he was in one leg stance increased. This indicated that he still lacked adequate motor control around the hip joint.

- The hypertonicity in the right iliocostalis lumborum, piriformis, ischiococcygeus and small external rotators of the hip and right IO had improved significantly.

- On assessment of the deep muscle system the patient demonstrated an isolated contraction of the PFM which resulted in a coordinated co-contraction of TrA and lumbosacral multifidus bilaterally.

As the motor control of deep muscles of the region was normalizing (at least in low loading situations), the focus of treatment turned towards integration of the deep and superficial muscle systems during functional activities, and vertical loading situations. Specifically, the patient was progressed through a graduated exercise programme based on the concepts of maintaining a submaximal co-contraction of the deep muscle system while holding postures and controlling motion that required superficial muscle activity. This was done first in stable, predictable situations and progressed to less stable, unpredictable and higher demand tasks. Due to the specific needs of this patient, special attention was given to disassociating the right leg from the trunk, and repetitive vertical loading. In time (approximately three months from the initial visit) this patient was able to control loading of the right side of his pelvis under high loading situations, and was able to return to his recreational activities (discharge RM 2/24).

DISCUSSION

As highlighted in Chapter 5, effective motor control training can only occur once a neurophysiological environment that is conducive to such training has been fashioned through sound clinical reasoning. Initially, any chemical inflammation or hypomobility secondary to joint and neuromeningeal components must be identified and treated. Concurrent with this, hypertonicity associated with protective splinting responses and compensatory recruitment patterns by the regional musculature must be minimized. Accomplishing these first two steps provides an opportunity to restore a neutral spinal posture and an optimal pattern of respiration (excluding the absence of any respiratory dysfunction or disease). In this particular case, decompression of the right sacroiliac joint was achieved through a high-velocity, low-amplitude (manipulation) manual therapy technique, and dry needling to the muscles that were creating excessive posterior compression (superficial erector spinae, piriformis, small external rotators of the hip as well as the gluteal) as well as the right IO. Neuromeningeal mobilizations and breathing exercises, as well as self-release and relaxation techniques aimed at restoring a resting neutral spine and femoral head position were also employed.

Once all sources of inflammation as well as joint and neuromeningeal restrictions have been eliminated, the deficits in the neuromuscular control of the deep muscle system can be identified and addressed. Up until this point in the rehabilitation process USI is incorporated primarily as an assessment and educational tool, providing the patient with information regarding the specific nature of their dysfunction. However, once motor control training begins it can augment the clinical skills that therapists already possess, and provide incomparable visual information upon which feedback, knowledge of results and knowledge of performance can be provided to the patient. In this particular scenario USI allowed for the assessment and facilitation of a group of muscles (PFM) that is virtually inaccessible to most manual therapists. Perhaps even more valuable was that it provided the patient with evidence of his dysfunction, as well as tangible feedback during the initial retraining stages of the PFM motor control so that he could disassociate them from abdominal wall straining. It is imperative to remember that deficits of the deep muscle system are often driven by augmented motor control of the regional superficial muscles (Richardson et al 2004). Thus, treatment may require down training techniques aimed at these superficial muscles as opposed to facilitation of the deep muscle in question. This point was clearly demonstrated in this case presentation with the persisting dominance of the right IO.

It is only after these steps, and when a coordinated co-contraction of the deep muscle system muscles can be generated and held by the patient, independent of feedback provided by the therapist or the technology, that loading of the region can occur. It is beyond the scope of this case presentation to provide a detailed description of this later stage of rehabilitation and the reader is referred elsewhere (Lee 2004, Richardson et al 2004). Although the focus of this later phase is the coordination of the deep and superficial muscles into functional activities, it is important that the subtle isolated deep muscle system contraction be continued, and revisited at each progression. This will assist the patient to prevent prematurely reverting to a bracing or rigidity motor control strategy when encountering slightly higher loads. The underlying concept is to encourage the muscles (both deep and superficial) to contract at the correct time, to the appropriate magnitude and duration for the task, and then relax to an appropriate level once the demand is removed. Numerous techniques can be used to implement this treatment strategy; those presented here are just one example, as it is not the technique that is important, rather the order and specificity with which each issue is addressed.

CONCLUSION

The appropriate use of USI can enhance the rehabilitation of lumbopelvic dysfunction. The challenge for the clinician is to determine when and in what form it should be integrated into the rehabilitation process. By presenting a practical illustration of the use of USI in the management of a specific patient it is hoped that the principles outlined in Chapter 5 take on greater meaning, and ultimately that clinicians will be encouraged to integrate USI into their practice.

APPENDIX D
Glossary

Absorption – In the context of ultrasound imaging, absorption refers to the transfer of energy from a sound wave to the surrounding tissues.

Acoustic shadowing – Refers to the reduction of the sound wave echo from structures that lie behind a strongly reflecting or attenuating structure (e.g. bone).

ALARA – An acronym for 'as low as reasonably achievable'. This is a principle governing the prudent use of ultrasound imaging which encourages gathering the most amount of information with the least amount of exposure. Specifically, this involves reducing exposure times, as well as lowering power output in favour of increased gain settings.

Anechoic – A material that does not produce echoes (e.g. ultrasound waves are allowed to pass through it). The more anechoic a structure or substance is, the darker it will appear within an ultrasound image.

Artefact – Refers to incorrect representations of anatomy or motion (e.g. situations that result in structures that are not real, missing, improperly located, or of inaccurate brightness,

shape or size). Examples include acoustic shadowing, edge shadowing and enhancement.

Attenuation – Defined as the reduction in the intensity or amplitude of a sound wave. Attenuation is expressed in decibels (dB) and it is caused by absorption, scattering and reflection of the sound wave as it travels. As attenuation increases, penetration decreases.

B mode – Brightness or brilliance mode.

Capnograph – An instrument that collects and analyses the carbon dioxide content in expired air.

Cavitation – Refers to the production and behaviour of gas bubbles within a liquid when exposed to a sound wave. This behaviour can be variable (e.g. oscillation or collapse) and depends upon factors such as the size of the cavity, and the nature of the immediate environment (Nyborg 2001).

Cine-loop – sequential display of all the ultrasound frames stored in the memory of an ultrasound unit at a controllable frame rate (Kremkau 2002).

Diagnostic ultrasound – Pertains to the use of ultrasound imaging to establish the nature of an injury or disease process. Diagnostic ultrasound units produce sound waves that enter the body and reflect off tissue interfaces. These reflections are subsequently collected and used to generate an image.

Echogenic – A structure or material that produces echoes (e.g. reflection of ultrasound waves). The more echogenic a structure or substance is, the whiter it will appear within an ultrasound image.

Edge shadowing – A type of artefact in which there is a reduction in the sound wave echo from a structure that is located in the shadow generated when a sound wave bends around a fluid-filled structure (e.g. bladder).

Enhancement – A type of artefact in which there is a strengthening of a sound wave echo distal to a weakly attenuating structure (e.g. a fluid-filled organ such as the bladder) (Kremkau 2002).

Far-field – The bottom half of the ultrasound screen, which represents that part of the body furthest from the ultrasound probe.

Feedback – Information provided by the various sensory organs (eyes, ears, nose, mouth, proprioceptive organs, thermal receptors etc.) before, during and after a task (Salmoni et al 1984).

Force closure – Refers to compression produced by the coordinated efforts of muscle, ligament, and fascia to augment the structure, orientation, and shape of a joint so that optimal load transfer can occur (Vleeming et al 1997, Lee 2004).

Form closure – Refers to how a joint's structure, orientation and shape contribute to load transfer (Vleeming et al 1997).

Frequency – The number of oscillations a molecule or a sound wave undergoes in one second. Frequency is expressed in units called hertz (Hz). 1 Hz = 1 cycle per second, 1 kHz = 1000 cycles

per second, and 1 MHz = 1,000,000 cycles per second.

Gain – In the context of ultrasound imaging, gain refers to the amount of amplification (expressed in decibels, dB) imparted to the electrical signal (which represents the echo from the tissues) coming from the transducer. The degree of amplification can be manipulated by the operator.

Global system – An anatomical term used to group muscles that are superficially placed. In the lumbopelvic region these muscles are torque producing and are responsible for controlling spinal orientation, as well as actively transferring load between the thoracic cage and pelvis (Bergmark 1989).

Hyperechoic – A structure or substance that is more echogenic, therefore whiter and brighter on the ultrasound screen, than surrounding tissue. The surface of bone and dense fascia are examples of hyperechoic media.

Hypocapnia – Defined as a reduction or deficiency in the arterial partial pressure of carbon dioxide. It is a result of behavioural, physical and/or environmental factors that lead to overbreathing, or ventilation in excess of metabolic need. The exaggerated respiratory response results in the elimination of carbon dioxide in volumes greater than it is being produced by the body and ultimately its deficiency. It is associated with respiratory alkalosis and a wide variety of symptoms, most notably paresthesia, increased resting muscle tone, dizziness, fatigue and chest pain (Gardner 1996).

Hypoechoic – A structure or substance that is less echogenic, therefore darker on the ultrasound screen, than surrounding tissue. Fluids such as blood and urine are examples of hypoechoic media.

Impedance – The impedance of a medium is equal to the density of that medium multiplied by its propagation speed. It is measured in rayls. The impedance of a medium increases if either the density or the propagation speed increase (Kremkau 2002).

Incidence angle – The angle between the sound coming from the transducer (incident sound) and a line perpendicular to the boundary of a medium (Kremkau 2002).

Instrument – In the context of ultrasound imaging, this is an electronic system that electrically drives a transducer, receives returning echoes, and presents them on a visual display as an anatomical image (Kremkau 2002).

Intensity – The rate at which energy is delivered per unit area. The intensity of an ultrasound wave is determined by the total power output of the probe (watts) divided by its area (cm^2) and is expressed in units of milliwatts per square centimetre (mW/cm^2).

Isoechoic – A structure or substance that is just as echogenic as, and therefore indistinguishable from, surrounding tissue.

Knowledge of performance – Information about the characteristics of a motor task (e.g. the task was performed too quickly or with too great of an effort) (Salmoni et al 1984).

Knowledge of results – Information provided after attempting a motor behaviour that tells the individual of their success in meeting a specific goal. Knowledge of results is in addition to the sources of feedback that are naturally available when an attempt at a motor task is made and is a verbal statement about the outcome of an attempt (successful vs. unsuccessful) as opposed to characteristics about the actual task (Salmoni et al 1984).

Linea alba – An anatomical term ('the white line') which refers to the vertical tendinous medial line seen along the anterior abdominal wall extending from the superior aspect of the symphysis pubis to the xyphoid. It is located between the inner or medial borders of the rectus abdominis muscles, and is formed by the blending of the aponeuroses of the oblique and transversus abdominal muscles (Williams 1995).

Linea semilunaris – An anatomical term ('the half curved line') which refers to the two vertical curved tendinous lines seen along the lateral aspect of the rectus abdominis muscles. Each line extends from the ninth rib to the pubic spine and is formed by the aponeuroses of the internal oblique at its point of division to enclose the rectus abdominis muscle. This aponeuroses is reinforced anteriorly by the fascia of the external oblique and posteriorly by the fascia of the transversus abdominis (Williams 1995).

Load transfer – Refers to the ability of a region of the body to transfer the loads that it is characteristically exposed to. For example, a primary function of the lumbopelvic region is to transfer the loads generated by body weight and gravity during standing, walking and sitting. How well the load is transferred dictates how efficient the region can function (Lee 2004).

Local system – An anatomical term used to describe a group of muscles which have their origin or insertion at the vertebrae (Bergmark 1989). These muscles are both anatomically and neurophysiologically suited to control intervertebral and intra-pelvic segmental mobility.

M mode – Motion mode, sometimes referred to as time-motion (TM) mode.

Motor control – Refers to patterning of muscle activation. Specifically, the timing, magnitude, sequence and relaxation of muscle activation.

Near-field – The top half of the ultrasound screen, which represents that part of the body closest to the ultra-sound probe.

Operating frequency – The preferred (maximum efficiency) frequency of operation of a transducer (Kremkau 2002). The operating frequency can also be referred to as the resonance or main frequency.

Penetration – In the context of ultra-sound imaging, penetration refers to the ability of sound to travel. Penetration is dependent upon the strength (intensity) and frequency of the sound wave as well as the compressibility of the medium that it travels through. For descriptive purposes, penetration refers to image depth.

Piezoelectric effect – Refers to a phenomenon in which some materials (ceramic, quartz etc.) produce a voltage or electrical current when deformed by an applied pressure such as sound (Kremkau 2002).

Pixel – A contraction of 'picture element'. A pixel refers to the smallest unit of a digitized, two dimensional image. A pixel can be described by its location (a set of x and y coordinates), as well as its brightness.

Probe – See transducer assembly.

Real-time ultrasound imaging (RTUS) – Refers to the rapid sequential display of ultrasound images resulting in a moving presentation (Kremkau 2002).

Reflection – As a sound wave propagates it breaks up (fractures) and loses its energy. Reflection is one form of fraction which refers to the portion of the sound wave that is reflected back towards the sound wave's original source. This reflected energy is what is captured and then used to generate an ultrasound image.

Refraction – Refers to the change in direction of a wave when it crosses a boundary. It comes from the modifica-tion of a Latin term meaning to turn aside.

Reliability (consistency) – Refers to the degree of stability of a measurement when it is repeated under identical conditions, or the degree to which a measure is free from random error. Inter-rater reliability refers to the degree of agreement between identical meas-urements taken by different individuals, while intra-rater reliability refers to the agreement of identical measurements taken by one individual at different points in time.

Resolution – The ability of an instru-ment to show detail.

Scan – Ultrasound lingo for a sono-graphic examination. Confusion can arise if used out of context as one may wonder whether a CT scan is being referred to as opposed to an ultrasound examination (Kremkau 2002).

Scatter – Describes the generation of secondary waves (fractions) in response to the primary sound wave encounter-ing a rough surface or heterogeneous media. Scattering is a type of artefact and is often referred to as diffusion.

Sonography – The term used to describe imaging resulting from ultrasound. Latin *sonus* (sound) and Greek *graphien* (to write).

Sound – Mechanical energy that propagates through air, water or any other matter in an orderly rhythmic fashion as determined by the molecular make-up of the transmitting medium.

Stress incontinence – The self-report or observation of urine leakage with physical exertion (Hay-Smith et al 2001).

Therapeutic ultrasound – Pertains to the use of ultrasound for therapeutic or healing purposes. In therapeutic applica-tions the mechanical and thermal effects of ultrasound on tissues are employed to promote changes within those tissues.

Unlike diagnostic applications, images of the tissues are not generated.

Transducer – Any device that converts one form of energy into another. The piezoelectric crystal is a transducer that converts electrical energy into sound energy and vice versa.

Transducer assembly (probe) – Consists of the transducer elements, their associated casing and dampening material.

Ultrasound – Sound with a frequency greater than what can be perceived by the human auditory system (>20,000 Hz).

Urge incontinence – The self-report or observation of involuntary urine leakage associated with a sudden, strong desire to void (Hay-Smith et al 2001).

Validity – Refers to the degree to which a test or procedure measures what it claims to measure.

Velocity – In the context of USI, velocity refers to the speed at which the vibratory motion is transmitted or propagated through a material.

Index

Page numbers marked with an asterisk★ refer to entries in the Glossary. Those in bold refer to illustrations.

177